Alan Bradley

The Art of Living Holistically
Balance and Purpose

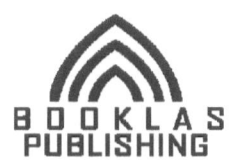

Original Title: The Art of Living Holistically
Copyright © 2023 by Luiz Antonio dos Santos
All rights reserved to Booklas.com
This book is intended for personal and spiritual development. The information and practices described are based on studies, traditional knowledge, and the experiences of authors and experts in the field. This content is not a substitute for medical advice or conventional therapies, serving as a complementary resource for well-being and personal growth.

Production Team
Editor: Luiz Antonio dos Santos
Text Revision: Clara Mendes, João Fernandes, Beatriz Lima
Graphic Design and Layout: Helena Castro
Cover Design: Booklas Studio / Lucas Silva

Publication and Identification
The Art of Living Holistically / By Luiz Antonio dos Santos
Booklas, 2024
Categories: Personal Development. Spirituality. Holism.
I. Silva, Lucas. II. Castro, Helena. III. Title.
DDC: 158.1
CDU: 159.9

All Rights Reserved
Booklas Publishing
José Delalíbera Street, 962
86.183-550 – Cambé – PR
Email: support@booklas.com
www.booklas.com

Summary

Prologue 5
Chapter 1 Holistic Introduction 7
Chapter 2 Integral Health 11
Chapter 3 Contemporary Spirituality 15
Chapter 4 Conscious Nutrition 19
Chapter 5 Holistic Sustainability 23
Chapter 6 Energy Therapies 28
Chapter 7 The Power of the Mind 32
Chapter 8 Conscious Relationships 36
Chapter 9 Purposeful Work 41
Chapter 10 Meditation and Silence 46
Chapter 11 Holistic Education 50
Chapter 12 The Inner Universe 54
Chapter 13 The Energy of Love 58
Chapter 14 Holism in Technology 62
Chapter 15 Resilience and Balance 67
Chapter 16 The Inner Journey 72
Chapter 17 Vibrations and Frequencies 76
Chapter 18 Science and Holism 81
Chapter 19 Connection with Nature 86
Chapter 20 Healing Through Sound 90
Chapter 21 The Power of Gratitude 94
Chapter 22 Rhythms and Cycles 98
Chapter 23 Emotions and Energy 102

Chapter 24 Radical Self-Acceptance 106
Chapter 25 Simplicity and Essence.. 110
Chapter 26 Global Connection... 114
Chapter 27 Awakening Consciousness 119
Chapter 28 Harmony in Spaces.. 123
Chapter 29 Ancestral Practices 127
Chapter 30 Life Purpose 131
Chapter 31 Holistic Spirituality in Childhood 135
Chapter 32 Energetic Communication 139
Chapter 33 Balancing Masculine and Feminine Energies 144
Chapter 34 Spiritual Reconnection 148
Chapter 35 Transcendence of the Ego 152
Chapter 36 Energetic Connection 156
Chapter 37 Synchronicity and Signs... 161
Chapter 38 Intuition and Wisdom 165
Chapter 39 Holism and Modernity.. 169
Chapter 40 Nocturnal Practices... 174
Chapter 41 Transgenerational Healing 178
Chapter 42 Collective Energy 182
Chapter 43 The Hero's Journey 186
Chapter 44 Expansion of Consciousness 190
Chapter 45 Time and the Present Moment................................. 194
Chapter 46 Holistic Leadership... 198
Chapter 47 Personal Alchemy.. 202
Chapter 48 Union and Integration.. 206
Chapter 49 The Holistic Future.. 210
Epilogue 214

Prologue

Life is not an isolated event; it is a continuous dance of connections and cycles. Every thought, every choice, and every experience are threads interwoven into a larger fabric, a unity often elusive to perception. Between the chaos of daily life and the quiet moments subtly calling for attention lies an unwavering truth: everything is interconnected.

The human gaze often seeks fragments, categorizing what it sees into parts and labels. Yet, there is something greater than the individual pieces—a harmony that emerges when the mind, body, spirit, and surrounding environment align. This vision, often called holistic, is not new. It resonates in the ancestral wisdom of those who lived in deep harmony with the rhythms of the earth and is renewed in modern science rediscovering the invisible symphony sustaining the universe.

The essence of holistic living does not lie in complexity but in integration. The body reflects the mind; the mind nourishes emotions; emotions resonate in energy; and energy echoes in the environment. To nurture one aspect while neglecting the others is like attempting to harmonize a melody while ignoring the balance of its notes. Health, purpose, and well-being emerge only when coherence exists among the parts that form the whole.

The paths to this coherence are diverse. Some are found in the profound silence of meditation, where the mind rests and reveals its hidden nuances. Others emerge in the simplicity of a meal prepared with awareness, where flavors not only nourish the body but celebrate a connection with the earth. There are also those moments when the simple act of walking among trees or observing the flow of a river awakens the realization that nature is not a backdrop but an extension of existence itself.

The practice of mindfulness offers a bridge to this integration. When the haste that fragments is abandoned, perception expands. A single breath can become a portal to the present, revealing that the now contains all that is needed. In this state of presence, even the challenges of daily life transform into opportunities for growth and balance.

Holism invites a broader perspective, where individual choices cease to be merely personal and become universal. An act as small as reducing waste or cultivating gratitude resonates in the collective because each gesture carries the potential to influence the larger web of life. Personal balance is reflected in a more harmonious world.

This journey is not linear. It is a continuous process of observation, practice, and learning. At times, the answers will seem clear; at others, more questions will arise. This dynamic is natural because living holistically is not about reaching a final state but adopting a conscious approach that evolves over time.

Within this space lies an invitation to explore not only the surface but the depths of oneself and the world. The proposition is clear: recognize the interconnections, integrate what is fragmented, and rediscover the full potential of what it means to live holistically.

Chapter 1
Holistic Introduction

Holism is not merely a philosophy; it is a way of perceiving the universe as an intricate and interconnected web. At its core, holism embraces the idea that every element of existence is woven into a greater tapestry where the whole is far more significant than the sum of its parts. This perspective, born from ancient wisdom and now resonating in modern life, challenges the fragmented view of the world that dominates contemporary thought.

The term "holism" originates from the Greek word *holos*, meaning "whole." It emerged in modern terminology in the early 20th century through the work of South African statesman and philosopher Jan Smuts. However, its essence predates written history, flowing through the veins of indigenous traditions, ancient spiritual systems, and the natural rhythms of life. Smuts defined holism as the principle of the whole being primary and unifying, influencing and shaping its components. This idea echoes deeply in cultures where the connection between body, mind, spirit, and environment forms the foundation of existence.

The holistic perspective contrasts sharply with reductionism, a framework that dissects phenomena into isolated parts to study them individually. While reductionism has contributed greatly to scientific advancements, it often overlooks the dynamic interplay between components. Holism, on the other hand, sees health, spirituality, relationships, and even societal structures as interconnected entities, thriving only when their intrinsic bonds are nurtured.

The modern world is witnessing a resurgence of this ancient worldview. From healthcare to environmental sustainability, and from personal development to technology, holism is shaping the way we interact with ourselves and our surroundings. The once-fringe ideas of interconnectedness and balance are now becoming central to how individuals and societies function. This transformation is not coincidental; it reflects a collective yearning to reconnect with what truly matters.

In health, holistic approaches recognize the intricate links between physical conditions, emotional states, and spiritual well-being. Practices such as yoga, meditation, and acupuncture embody this principle, treating individuals as whole beings rather than merely addressing isolated symptoms. In spirituality, the holistic lens transcends religious dogma, embracing mindfulness, energy work, and universal connection as pathways to personal and collective awakening.

Relationships, too, are enriched by this perspective. Empathy, active listening, and authentic communication thrive when seen through the lens of holism, where every interaction contributes to the larger relational dynamic. Communities, workplaces, and even global movements reflect this interconnectedness, recognizing that individual actions ripple outward to affect the collective fabric of humanity.

This integrative way of living is particularly evident in how people approach daily life. The rise of practices like slow living, minimalism, and eco-consciousness signals a shift away from consumption-driven existence toward purposeful engagement with the world. Whether through sustainable eating habits, mindfulness exercises, or cultivating gratitude, the holistic path offers tools to rediscover harmony in an often chaotic world.

Historically, holistic principles have thrived in systems like Traditional Chinese Medicine, Ayurveda, and indigenous healing practices. These frameworks have always prioritized balance—be it between the elements, energies, or the individual and their environment. Today, these principles are re-emerging not as relics of the past but as profound guides for the future. As science begins to validate the efficacy of these practices, the gap between ancient wisdom and modern understanding is narrowing.

Yet, holism is not confined to health and personal development. Its principles extend to how we interact with technology, nature, and the cosmos itself. Consider how ecological practices emphasize biodiversity, a holistic acknowledgment that every species contributes to the planet's equilibrium. Similarly, advancements in quantum physics reveal a universe where particles are interconnected, mirroring the ancient belief in a unified existence.

The resurgence of the holistic approach signals a turning point for humanity. It is an invitation to rediscover the innate wisdom within ourselves and to align with the rhythms of the world around us. As the digital age accelerates, many are finding solace in practices that reconnect them to the tangible, the present, and the transcendent. Holism is not a rejection of progress but a reminder to advance with awareness and intention.

In understanding the essence of holism, one must also consider the inner journey it demands. To live holistically is to cultivate awareness, to honor the connections between thought and action, and to recognize the sacred interplay of individuality and unity. It asks for a willingness to explore the self deeply, to embrace contradictions, and to seek harmony in diversity.

Modern life, with its relentless pace and distractions, often pulls individuals away from this sense of connection. Yet, the holistic perspective offers an antidote—a pathway back to wholeness. By weaving practices such as mindfulness, intentional living, and conscious interaction into daily routines, one can begin to experience the profound impact of living holistically. It is not merely about personal fulfillment; it is about contributing to a world where balance and unity prevail.

Holism also challenges traditional paradigms of success, urging individuals to measure their lives not by external achievements but by the depth of their connections, the harmony of their existence, and the authenticity of their actions. This shift is not about abandoning ambition but aligning it with values that nurture both the self and the world.

The integration of holistic principles into daily life is not an endpoint but a continuous journey. It evolves with each individual, adapting to their unique needs and aspirations. Whether through the quiet stillness of meditation, the active engagement of community service, or the transformative power of introspection, the holistic path unfolds as a deeply personal and profoundly universal experience.

As society embraces this ancient yet ever-relevant perspective, the ripple effects are transformative. The holistic mindset fosters empathy, sustainability, and innovation, enabling individuals to thrive while contributing to a greater good. It is a call to remember that we are not separate from the world around us but intrinsic to its unfolding story.

Through holism, the fragmented pieces of existence are woven into a coherent and meaningful whole. It is a lens through which to view life not as a series of disconnected moments but as an evolving journey of unity, balance, and purpose. The holistic way of living is not merely an alternative; it is an essential framework for navigating the complexities of the modern era while honoring the timeless truths of our existence.

Chapter 2
Integral Health

Health is more than the absence of illness. It is a dynamic state of harmony that encompasses physical vitality, emotional resilience, mental clarity, and spiritual alignment. Integral health emerges from the recognition that every aspect of our being is interconnected, and true wellness cannot exist in isolation. The holistic approach to health embraces this understanding, offering a path that integrates ancient wisdom with modern practices to achieve balance and well-being.

For centuries, traditional systems of medicine like Ayurveda, Traditional Chinese Medicine, and indigenous healing practices have viewed health through a holistic lens. These systems emphasize harmony within the body and with the external environment, offering tools and rituals to nurture equilibrium. In Ayurveda, for instance, the concept of *doshas*—energetic forces that govern the body—guides individualized treatments to restore balance. Traditional Chinese Medicine, with its focus on *qi* (vital energy), highlights the flow of energy through meridians and its role in maintaining health.

Modern medicine, with its groundbreaking discoveries and life-saving technologies, has transformed how we address illness. However, it often focuses on symptoms rather than root causes. The rise of integrative medicine—a field that combines conventional treatments with holistic approaches—reflects a growing acknowledgment that healing must address the whole person. Practices like yoga, meditation, and acupuncture, once seen as alternative, are now recognized as powerful tools to complement medical treatments.

Yoga, a practice with origins in ancient India, exemplifies the essence of integral health. It is not merely a physical exercise but a union of body, mind, and spirit. The deliberate movement of asanas (poses), the rhythm of breath, and the meditative focus create a state of coherence within the practitioner. Yoga reduces stress, enhances flexibility, and cultivates mindfulness, enabling individuals to connect with their inner selves.

Meditation, another cornerstone of holistic health, offers profound benefits for mental clarity and emotional stability. By quieting the mind, meditation allows the practitioner to observe thoughts without judgment, fostering self-awareness and reducing anxiety. Scientific studies reveal that regular meditation reduces cortisol levels, improves immune function, and even alters brain structure in ways that promote resilience and focus.

Therapies such as acupuncture and Reiki address the energetic dimensions of health. Acupuncture, rooted in Traditional Chinese Medicine, stimulates specific points along the body's meridians to enhance the flow of energy. This practice alleviates pain, reduces inflammation, and balances the nervous system. Reiki, an energy healing technique, uses gentle touch or intention to harmonize the body's vibrational field, promoting relaxation and self-healing.

Integral health also emphasizes the role of nutrition in well-being. Holistic nutrition views food as medicine, recognizing its ability to nourish not just the body but the mind and spirit. Whole, unprocessed foods rich in vitamins, minerals, and life force energy form the foundation of this approach. Beyond calories and nutrients, the vibrational quality of food—its freshness, source, and preparation—affects the individual's energy and vitality.

The relationship between emotional health and physical health is undeniable. Stress, unresolved trauma, and negative emotions manifest in the body as tension, illness, or chronic conditions. Holistic practices encourage the release of emotional blockages through methods like journaling, therapy, or expressive arts. These practices create space for healing, allowing individuals to process and transform their emotional experiences.

Case studies illustrate the transformative power of integral health. Consider the story of a woman battling chronic fatigue syndrome. Conventional medicine offered symptom management, but true healing came when she adopted a holistic approach. Through yoga, a nutrient-dense diet, and energy healing sessions, she regained her vitality and reconnected with her purpose. Her journey demonstrates that addressing the whole person—body, mind, and spirit—can lead to profound recovery.

Holistic health also fosters community and connection. Group yoga classes, meditation circles, and wellness retreats create spaces where individuals can share their journeys and support one another. This sense of belonging enhances healing, as the emotional bonds formed within these communities provide strength and encouragement.

In the fast-paced modern world, burnout has become a common affliction. Integral health offers a way to combat this by teaching individuals to listen to their bodies, set boundaries, and prioritize self-care. Practices like mindful breathing, nature walks, and digital detoxes restore balance and prevent the depletion of energy reserves.

The workplace, too, is embracing holistic health. Companies now offer mindfulness programs, wellness challenges, and access to integrative therapies to support employee well-being. These initiatives recognize that a healthy workforce is not only more productive but also more creative and engaged.

Holistic health is not a one-size-fits-all approach. It honors the uniqueness of each individual, encouraging personalized practices that align with their needs and preferences. Whether through morning meditations, evening journaling, or weekend hikes, the path to integral health is as diverse as those who walk it.

The ripple effects of adopting integral health extend beyond the individual. Families thrive when members prioritize well-being and support one another's practices. Communities grow stronger as individuals share their experiences and knowledge. Even the environment benefits, as holistic health often inspires sustainable living and mindful consumption.

Science continues to validate the principles of integral health. Studies on the gut-brain connection reveal how nutrition and mental health are intertwined. Research on the effects of mindfulness on chronic pain demonstrates the power of the mind to influence the body. These findings bridge the gap between ancient wisdom and modern understanding, offering a comprehensive view of health that is both timeless and innovative.

Integral health is a journey, not a destination. It invites individuals to explore their inner and outer worlds, to nurture their bodies and spirits, and to embrace a life of balance and harmony. By integrating holistic practices into daily routines, individuals can unlock their potential for vitality and joy.

In this interconnected web of existence, health is not an isolated phenomenon but a reflection of how we relate to ourselves, each other, and the world. The path to integral health is one of discovery, growth, and connection, where every step taken enriches the whole. It is a call to honor the sacredness of life and to embody the principles of harmony, unity, and love.

Chapter 3
Contemporary Spirituality

In a world increasingly disconnected from traditional religious frameworks, spirituality has taken on new forms, shedding dogma and embracing individuality. This contemporary approach to spirituality transcends institutional boundaries, offering a deeply personal and transformative connection to something greater than oneself. At its heart, it is about exploring the sacred in everyday life, nurturing a sense of purpose, and awakening to the profound interconnectedness of all existence.

The roots of contemporary spirituality lie in ancient practices, but its modern expression reflects the shifting needs and desires of today's seekers. While traditional religions often prescribe fixed paths, modern spirituality empowers individuals to forge their own journeys, guided by intuition, experience, and inner wisdom. This freedom has birthed a movement where mindfulness, meditation, and energy work coexist with scientific understanding, creating a bridge between the mystical and the tangible.

Mindfulness is a cornerstone of contemporary spirituality. Originating from Buddhist teachings, mindfulness has been adapted into a secular practice accessible to all. It invites individuals to anchor themselves in the present moment, cultivating awareness and acceptance without judgment. This simple yet profound practice transforms mundane activities into opportunities for connection and insight. Washing dishes becomes a meditation on water and effort; walking in nature becomes a communion with the earth.

Meditation, closely tied to mindfulness, has evolved into diverse forms that cater to different needs. From silent Vipassana retreats to guided visualizations, meditation serves as a tool to quiet the mind, access inner peace, and connect with the vastness within. Some use meditation to heal emotional wounds, others to expand their consciousness or align with their higher selves. Each path is valid, reflecting the deeply personal nature of modern spirituality.

The resurgence of energy work in contemporary spirituality highlights humanity's growing awareness of the unseen forces that shape our lives. Practices like Reiki, sound healing, and chakra balancing help individuals realign with their natural energetic flow. These techniques emphasize the idea that we are more than physical bodies; we are vibrational beings, influenced by the subtle energies of our thoughts, emotions, and surroundings.

Contemporary spirituality also embraces the concept of connection—not only to the divine but also to oneself, others, and the universe. This connection fosters a sense of belonging that transcends divisions of race, culture, or belief. It reminds us that we are threads in a vast, intricate tapestry, each contributing to the beauty and integrity of the whole.

In today's spiritual landscape, nature often becomes the sanctuary. The forest, the ocean, and the sky serve as places of worship where seekers find solace and inspiration. Practices like forest bathing, where individuals immerse themselves in the natural world, awaken a deep reverence for life. This communion with nature reinforces the awareness that spirituality is not confined to rituals or sacred texts; it is alive in the rustling of leaves, the rhythm of waves, and the vastness of the cosmos.

One of the hallmarks of contemporary spirituality is its inclusivity. It does not demand adherence to specific doctrines but encourages exploration. Many individuals draw from multiple traditions, creating a personal tapestry of beliefs and practices. A person might incorporate Buddhist meditation, Hindu mantras,

Christian prayer, and Native American rituals into their spiritual routine, finding resonance and meaning in the diversity.

The shift toward experiential spirituality also reflects a desire for authenticity. Modern seekers are less interested in theories and more drawn to practices that produce tangible results. They seek experiences that bring clarity, healing, and transformation. Whether through ecstatic dance, breathwork, or silent contemplation, these experiences create moments of transcendence where the boundaries of self dissolve, revealing a profound unity with the greater whole.

Contemporary spirituality also embraces the idea of purpose and meaning. For many, the spiritual path is not about escaping the world but engaging with it more fully. It inspires individuals to live with integrity, compassion, and intention, recognizing that every action contributes to the collective energy of the planet. This purpose-driven approach often leads to acts of service, environmental stewardship, and a commitment to social justice.

The integration of ancient practices with modern technology has further shaped contemporary spirituality. Apps for meditation, online communities for spiritual discussion, and virtual retreats offer new ways to connect and grow. Technology, often criticized for fostering disconnection, can also be a tool for deepening spiritual engagement when used mindfully. It allows for the global exchange of wisdom, making teachings once confined to specific cultures accessible to all.

Contemporary spirituality also challenges the notion of hierarchy in spiritual growth. It emphasizes that enlightenment is not reserved for gurus or mystics but is available to anyone willing to explore their inner world. Teachers and guides serve not as authorities but as companions on the journey, offering insights and tools while honoring the autonomy of the seeker.

The challenges of modern life—stress, disconnection, and existential uncertainty—have driven many toward this evolving spirituality. It provides a refuge where individuals can rediscover their inner strength, align with their values, and cultivate resilience. In this context, spirituality is not a luxury but a necessity, a lifeline that anchors us in a world of constant change.

Stories of transformation illustrate the power of contemporary spirituality. A man burdened by the pressures of corporate life finds peace through mindfulness, leading him to create a more balanced and fulfilling career. A woman grieving the loss of a loved one discovers solace in energy healing, helping her to process her emotions and embrace a renewed sense of purpose. These journeys reveal that spirituality is not about escaping life's challenges but embracing them as catalysts for growth.

This modern spiritual movement is not without its critics. Some view it as superficial or commodified, pointing to the commercialization of practices like yoga or the proliferation of self-help products. However, these critiques highlight the need for discernment and authenticity in the spiritual journey. True spirituality transcends trends and marketing, grounding itself in genuine connection and transformation.

Ultimately, contemporary spirituality is a reminder that the sacred is always present, waiting to be noticed. It calls us to awaken from the trance of routine and remember the wonder of existence. It invites us to see the divine in ourselves, each other, and the world around us.

In this unfolding narrative of spiritual evolution, there are no final answers, only deeper questions and richer experiences. Contemporary spirituality is not a fixed destination but a dynamic journey, a path that adapts to the ever-changing landscape of human consciousness. It is a testament to the resilience and creativity of the human spirit, continually seeking meaning, connection, and wholeness in an ever-expanding universe.

Chapter 4
Conscious Nutrition

Nutrition, in its truest form, transcends the simple act of feeding the body. It is an intricate relationship between the food we consume, the energy it provides, and the overall harmony it fosters within us. Conscious nutrition embodies this holistic perspective, emphasizing that our dietary choices influence not just our physical health, but also our mental clarity, emotional stability, and spiritual growth.

The roots of conscious nutrition lie in ancient traditions that viewed food as sacred. For centuries, cultures around the world recognized the energetic properties of what they ate, understanding that food carried life force, or *prana*, and could align the body with the rhythms of nature. In Ayurveda, foods are categorized by their effects on the body's doshas—balancing or aggravating these energies. Similarly, in Traditional Chinese Medicine, the thermal and energetic qualities of food are believed to affect the body's *qi* and internal harmony.

In the modern world, conscious nutrition has gained renewed importance. As processed and artificial foods dominate diets, people are increasingly turning to natural, whole, and sustainable alternatives. This movement is not just about returning to traditional practices; it's about reclaiming the power of food to heal, energize, and connect us to the earth.

A key aspect of conscious nutrition is mindfulness. Eating becomes a deliberate act, rooted in awareness and presence. Each meal is an opportunity to engage the senses, savor the flavors, and honor the source of sustenance. This practice counters the habit of unconscious eating, where meals are consumed hastily or distractedly, often leading to overeating and a disconnection from the body's signals.

Conscious nutrition also emphasizes the importance of understanding the origins of our food. Where was it grown? Who harvested it? How was it treated during its journey to our plate? These questions guide us toward ethical and sustainable choices. Organic produce, free-range animal products, and locally sourced ingredients reflect a commitment to quality and environmental stewardship. By choosing such foods, we align ourselves with practices that honor the planet and its ecosystems.

One of the pillars of conscious nutrition is the idea of eating for energy. Every food carries a vibrational quality that interacts with our body's energy field. Fresh fruits and vegetables, for example, are high-vibration foods, rich in nutrients and life force. In contrast, heavily processed foods, laden with chemicals and preservatives, are considered low-vibration and can deplete our energy. This awareness leads to choices that not only nourish the body but also elevate the mind and spirit.

The practice of intuitive eating is another hallmark of conscious nutrition. Intuitive eating invites us to listen to our bodies, trusting their wisdom to guide our food choices. Rather than adhering to rigid diets or external rules, this approach honors the body's natural hunger and satiety signals. It encourages us to ask questions like: What does my body need right now? How will this food make me feel? Over time, this practice fosters a deep connection to our inner selves, allowing us to cultivate a harmonious relationship with food.

In addition to the physical and energetic aspects, conscious nutrition considers the emotional dimensions of eating. Food is often intertwined with memories, culture, and comfort, and these associations can influence our dietary habits. By becoming aware of emotional triggers, such as stress or sadness, we can begin to untangle unhealthy patterns and create space for mindful choices.

Sustainability is another vital component of conscious nutrition. Our dietary decisions impact the planet in profound ways. Choosing plant-based meals, reducing food waste, and supporting regenerative farming practices are all steps toward a more sustainable future. Conscious eaters recognize that their plates are not isolated from the world but are deeply connected to the health of the environment.

The benefits of adopting conscious nutrition are vast and far-reaching. On a physical level, it promotes optimal digestion, sustained energy, and a strengthened immune system. Mentally, it enhances focus and clarity, while emotionally, it cultivates a sense of balance and contentment. Spiritually, it deepens our connection to the earth and reminds us of the sacredness of nourishment.

Examples of this transformative approach abound. A woman struggling with chronic digestive issues finds relief through mindful eating and a diet centered on whole foods. A man seeking greater vitality discovers the power of green smoothies, packed with nutrient-dense ingredients that rejuvenate his energy. Families who embrace sustainable practices, such as growing their own vegetables or composting, experience a newfound appreciation for the cycle of life.

Cultural practices around food also offer inspiration for conscious nutrition. The Japanese concept of *hara hachi bu*, which encourages eating until one is 80% full, promotes moderation and respect for the body's needs. The Mediterranean diet, with its emphasis on fresh produce, olive oil, and communal meals, exemplifies the joy of sharing food in a mindful and balanced way. Indigenous traditions often view food as medicine, fostering reverence for the plants and animals that sustain life.

Rituals can further enhance the practice of conscious nutrition. Taking a moment of gratitude before a meal, for instance, sets an intention of mindfulness and appreciation. Preparing food with care, using fresh ingredients and simple techniques, transforms cooking into a meditative act. Even small adjustments, like eating without distractions or chewing slowly, can have a profound impact on how we experience and digest our meals.

Challenges inevitably arise on the journey toward conscious nutrition. The convenience of fast food, the allure of sugary treats, and the pressures of modern life can make it difficult to maintain mindful eating habits. However, the holistic perspective emphasizes progress over perfection. Each mindful choice, no matter how small, contributes to a broader shift in consciousness.

The integration of conscious nutrition into daily life is not about restriction or deprivation. Instead, it is about abundance—the abundance of flavors, nutrients, and connection that food can provide. It is an invitation to explore, experiment, and rediscover the joy of eating.

In the grander scheme, conscious nutrition reflects a deeper truth: that we are not separate from the earth or its cycles. The food we eat becomes part of us, linking us to the soil, the sun, and the water that nurtured it. This awareness transforms eating into a sacred act, a reminder of our place within the interconnected web of life.

By embracing conscious nutrition, we nourish not only our bodies but also our spirits, fostering a relationship with food that is grounded in respect, gratitude, and love. It is a journey of self-discovery, a celebration of the earth's gifts, and a step toward a more harmonious existence. Through mindful and intentional eating, we align ourselves with the rhythms of nature, creating a foundation of balance and vitality that sustains us in all aspects of life.

Chapter 5
Holistic Sustainability

Holistic sustainability is a philosophy that transcends mere environmental conservation. It is a way of life that integrates mindful consumption, respect for natural resources, and a deep awareness of the interconnectedness of all living systems. While sustainability often focuses on reducing carbon footprints and preserving ecosystems, the holistic approach extends further, weaving in emotional, spiritual, and social dimensions. It asks not just what we can do to protect the earth, but how we can live in harmony with it, fostering balance within ourselves and the planet.

At the heart of holistic sustainability lies the recognition that humanity is not separate from nature but an integral part of it. Ancient cultures understood this intuitively, embedding practices of reverence for the earth into their daily lives. Indigenous traditions, for example, view land as sacred, treating it not as a commodity to be exploited but as a partner to be cared for. These traditions emphasize reciprocity—taking only what is needed and giving back in gratitude.

Modern society, with its rapid industrialization and consumerism, has largely severed this connection. Holistic sustainability seeks to bridge the gap, offering a pathway to reconnect with nature while addressing the urgent ecological crises of our time. It begins with a shift in mindset: from seeing the earth as a resource to be extracted to honoring it as a living, breathing entity that sustains all life.

Mindful consumption is a cornerstone of holistic sustainability. It involves questioning the origins, production, and impact of the goods we use. Every product we buy, every meal we eat, and every choice we make has an ecological footprint. By choosing locally sourced, ethically produced, and minimally packaged items, we reduce waste and support practices that align with environmental stewardship. For example, opting for reusable items, such as water bottles and shopping bags, minimizes single-use plastics that pollute oceans and harm wildlife.

Another key aspect is the practice of reducing, reusing, and recycling, often referred to as the "three R's." While recycling is widely promoted, reduction and reuse are equally, if not more, important. Reducing consumption limits the demand for resources, while reusing extends the lifespan of items, preventing them from becoming waste. These practices encourage creativity and innovation, transforming discarded materials into functional or artistic objects.

Holistic sustainability also encompasses energy use. Renewable energy sources, such as solar, wind, and hydroelectric power, offer alternatives to fossil fuels, reducing greenhouse gas emissions and mitigating climate change. On a personal level, small changes like using energy-efficient appliances, turning off lights, and insulating homes contribute to a more sustainable lifestyle.

Food plays a central role in holistic sustainability. Industrial agriculture, with its heavy reliance on chemicals, monocropping, and deforestation, is one of the leading contributors to environmental degradation. By supporting organic and regenerative farming, individuals can help restore soil health, preserve biodiversity, and reduce pollution. Consuming more plant-based meals further reduces the environmental impact, as livestock farming requires vast amounts of land, water, and energy.

Water conservation is another critical element. Freshwater is a finite resource, and its overuse threatens ecosystems and human communities alike. Simple actions, like fixing leaks, installing low-flow fixtures, and harvesting rainwater, make a significant difference. Holistic sustainability encourages viewing water not as a utility but as a sacred source of life, deserving care and protection.

Community engagement amplifies the impact of individual efforts. Holistic sustainability thrives in collective actions, where people come together to plant trees, clean beaches, or establish community gardens. These initiatives not only benefit the environment but also strengthen social bonds and foster a sense of shared responsibility. When communities embrace sustainable practices, they create ripple effects that inspire broader cultural shifts.

Holistic sustainability also addresses the emotional and spiritual connection to the earth. Spending time in nature—whether hiking through forests, meditating by rivers, or simply tending to a garden—rekindles this bond. These moments of connection remind us of the beauty and abundance of the natural world, inspiring gratitude and a deeper commitment to its preservation.

Education plays a crucial role in cultivating sustainable mindsets. Teaching children about the importance of ecosystems, biodiversity, and environmental ethics lays the foundation for future generations to live in harmony with the planet. Schools that incorporate sustainability into their curricula encourage students to think critically about their impact and explore innovative solutions to ecological challenges.

Technology, often viewed as a source of environmental harm, can also be a powerful ally in holistic sustainability. Smart systems that monitor energy use, apps that track carbon footprints, and platforms that promote eco-friendly products demonstrate how innovation can support sustainable living. However, the holistic perspective reminds us to balance technological advancement with simplicity, ensuring that progress serves the greater good.

One inspiring example of holistic sustainability in action is the zero-waste movement. Individuals and communities committed to producing no waste adopt practices like composting, bulk shopping, and repurposing items. These efforts challenge conventional consumption habits, proving that it is possible to live lightly on the earth without sacrificing comfort or convenience.

Another example is the rise of permaculture, a design philosophy that mimics natural ecosystems to create self-sustaining environments. Permaculture gardens produce food, conserve water, and build soil fertility, embodying the principles of holistic sustainability. These gardens often serve as models for sustainable agriculture, inspiring others to adopt regenerative practices.

The fashion industry, a major polluter, is also undergoing a transformation. Sustainable fashion brands are prioritizing ethical labor practices, organic materials, and circular design, where garments are recycled or biodegradable. By choosing quality over quantity and supporting such brands, consumers contribute to a more sustainable future.

Holistic sustainability extends beyond environmental actions to encompass social and economic dimensions. Fair trade practices, for instance, ensure that workers receive fair wages and safe working conditions, fostering equity and well-being. Supporting local businesses strengthens communities, reduces transportation emissions, and promotes a circular economy where resources remain in use for as long as possible.

The challenges of adopting holistic sustainability are real. Convenience, habit, and systemic barriers often hinder change. However, the holistic perspective encourages a mindset of progress, not perfection. Each small step—whether planting a tree, reducing food waste, or switching to renewable energy—contributes to the larger goal of planetary balance.

Holistic sustainability is not a trend but a necessary evolution. It is a call to reimagine our relationship with the earth, shifting from exploitation to stewardship. It reminds us that every action, no matter how small, has an impact and that collective efforts can create profound change.

In embracing holistic sustainability, we honor the interconnected web of life. We acknowledge that our well-being is inseparable from the health of the planet and that by nurturing the earth, we nurture ourselves. This philosophy invites us to live with intention, gratitude, and responsibility, creating a world where humanity and nature thrive together.

Chapter 6
Energy Therapies

Beneath the surface of what we perceive as physical lies an intricate web of energy that animates and sustains all life. Energy therapies, rooted in ancient traditions and increasingly embraced in modern practices, tap into this unseen realm to promote healing and balance. These therapies recognize that disturbances in the body's energetic field can manifest as physical illness, emotional unrest, or mental disarray, and they seek to harmonize these energies to restore well-being.

Energy therapies are grounded in the belief that we are not merely physical beings but dynamic systems of energy interconnected with the universe. From the *qi* of Traditional Chinese Medicine to the *prana* of Indian yoga, cultures worldwide have long understood the vital force that flows through us. These traditions teach that when this energy flows freely, we thrive; when it becomes blocked or stagnant, imbalance arises.

Modern science is beginning to validate these ancient concepts. Advances in quantum physics reveal that all matter is energy vibrating at different frequencies. This understanding bridges the gap between the mystical and the scientific, shedding light on how energy therapies work on both subtle and tangible levels.

Reiki, one of the most well-known energy therapies, originated in Japan and is now practiced globally. The word "Reiki" combines two Japanese words: *rei* (universal) and *ki* (life energy). Practitioners channel this universal energy through their hands, gently placing them on or near the recipient's body to facilitate healing. Reiki sessions often bring deep relaxation, reduce stress, and promote a sense of peace. While subtle, its effects can be profound, addressing not only physical discomfort but also emotional wounds and spiritual imbalances.

Another powerful modality is chakra therapy, which focuses on the body's seven main energy centers. Each chakra corresponds to specific physical, emotional, and spiritual aspects of life. When a chakra is blocked or overactive, it disrupts the flow of energy, leading to challenges in the associated areas. For example, an imbalanced heart chakra may manifest as difficulty in relationships, while a blocked throat chakra might hinder communication. Chakra therapy uses techniques such as visualization, affirmations, and sound healing to restore balance and vitality.

Sound healing, an ancient practice used by cultures worldwide, employs vibrations to align the body's energy field. Instruments such as singing bowls, tuning forks, and gongs produce frequencies that resonate with specific energetic patterns. These vibrations penetrate deeply, clearing blockages and recalibrating the body's natural rhythms. Tibetan singing bowls, for instance, are tuned to frequencies that harmonize with the chakras, while gongs create waves of sound that promote relaxation and emotional release.

Crystal healing is another therapy that taps into the vibrational properties of natural stones and minerals. Crystals are believed to carry specific energies that interact with the body's energetic field. Amethyst, for instance, is associated with calming and spiritual clarity, while rose quartz promotes love and emotional healing. Practitioners place crystals on or around the body, or individuals carry them as talismans to support specific intentions.

Acupuncture, rooted in Traditional Chinese Medicine, focuses on restoring the flow of *qi* through the body's meridians. By inserting fine needles into specific points, acupuncture stimulates the body's self-healing mechanisms. It is widely used to treat conditions such as chronic pain, anxiety, and digestive issues. Acupuncture's ability to regulate the nervous system and enhance energy flow demonstrates the profound connection between the physical and energetic realms.

Cupping therapy, often used alongside acupuncture, employs suction to release stagnation in the body's energy pathways. Glass or silicone cups are placed on the skin, creating a vacuum that draws blood and energy to the surface. This technique alleviates pain, reduces inflammation, and supports detoxification, allowing energy to circulate freely once again.

Energy therapies are not limited to professional practices; they can also be incorporated into daily life. Grounding, or earthing, is a simple yet effective way to harmonize one's energy with the earth's natural frequencies. Walking barefoot on grass, sand, or soil allows the body to absorb the earth's electrons, neutralizing stress and promoting physical and emotional balance.

Breathwork is another accessible practice that aligns the body's energy. By consciously controlling the breath, individuals can regulate their nervous system and enhance the flow of life force. Techniques such as *pranayama* (yogic breath control) and the Wim Hof Method demonstrate the transformative power of intentional breathing, helping to clear energetic blockages and elevate one's state of consciousness.

Visualization is yet another tool for energy alignment. By imagining light or specific colors flowing through the body, individuals can direct energy to areas that need healing. This practice taps into the mind's ability to influence the body, bridging the gap between thought and energetic reality.

Energy therapies often produce subtle, cumulative effects. While some may experience immediate shifts, others find that consistent practice is necessary to achieve lasting transformation. This process reflects the holistic principle that healing is a journey, not an instant fix.

Critics of energy therapies often point to the lack of scientific evidence for certain modalities. However, many practitioners argue that these therapies operate beyond the scope of conventional measurement tools, working in realms where intuition and experience take precedence over data. Moreover, as research into subtle energy fields advances, the scientific community is beginning to explore phenomena that were once dismissed as unquantifiable.

One notable study conducted on Reiki demonstrated its ability to reduce stress and improve quality of life in patients undergoing cancer treatment. Similarly, research on sound healing has shown that specific frequencies can reduce anxiety, lower heart rates, and enhance overall well-being. These findings, while preliminary, highlight the potential of energy therapies to complement conventional approaches to health.

Energy therapies also serve as a reminder of the body's innate wisdom and ability to heal. They encourage individuals to become active participants in their own well-being, fostering a sense of empowerment and self-awareness. By tuning into their energy, people can develop a deeper understanding of their needs and learn to navigate life's challenges with greater resilience.

Incorporating energy practices into everyday routines not only supports personal well-being but also contributes to collective harmony. When individuals align their energy, they radiate positivity, influencing their environment and the people around them. This ripple effect embodies the holistic principle that personal transformation contributes to universal balance.

Energy therapies are more than healing techniques; they are pathways to a deeper connection with oneself and the universe. They invite us to explore the unseen, to trust in the subtle, and to honor the vibrational essence of life. By embracing these practices, we open ourselves to new dimensions of well-being, cultivating harmony within and around us.

The journey into energy healing is one of discovery, where the tangible and intangible converge. It is an exploration of the infinite potential that resides within us and the boundless energy that surrounds us. Through these therapies, we step into a world where healing is not just physical but vibrational, offering profound transformation for the body, mind, and soul.

Chapter 7
The Power of the Mind

The mind is both a tool and a mystery—a force capable of shaping reality, directing emotions, and influencing the course of life itself. For the holistic individual, understanding and harnessing the power of the mind is essential to personal growth and transformation. This chapter delves into the extraordinary capabilities of the human mind, exploring how thoughts, beliefs, and intentions can create profound changes in health, relationships, and the spiritual journey.

At the heart of this exploration lies a simple yet profound truth: the mind is the architect of experience. Ancient philosophies have long held that reality is shaped not only by external circumstances but by perception. Modern science, particularly in the field of neuroplasticity, confirms this idea. The brain is not static; it changes and adapts based on thoughts, emotions, and repeated patterns of behavior. This means that by consciously directing the mind, individuals can rewire their brains, cultivate positive habits, and create new possibilities.

One of the most powerful tools for harnessing the mind's potential is visualization. By vividly imagining a desired outcome, the brain begins to interpret the visualization as reality, activating the neural pathways associated with the experience. Athletes, for instance, often use mental rehearsal to improve performance, visualizing every movement of their routines with precision. Similarly, individuals can use visualization to manifest goals, heal emotional wounds, or enhance creativity.

Closely tied to visualization is the practice of affirmation. Affirmations are positive, intentional statements that reprogram the subconscious mind. By repeating phrases like "I am worthy," "I attract abundance," or "I am healthy and strong," individuals replace limiting beliefs with empowering ones. This process, while simple, requires consistency and faith, as it challenges deep-seated mental patterns that may have been reinforced over years or even decades.

The power of thought is another cornerstone of mental mastery. Thoughts are not merely fleeting impulses; they carry energy and influence. Positive thoughts cultivate hope, motivation, and joy, while negative thoughts can spiral into fear, doubt, and despair. Recognizing the impact of thoughts, the holistic individual practices mindfulness to observe the mind without attachment. This allows them to interrupt unhelpful patterns and redirect their mental energy toward constructive and uplifting perspectives.

Meditation is perhaps the most transformative practice for developing mastery over the mind. By sitting in stillness and observing the flow of thoughts, practitioners gain insight into their mental processes. Meditation creates a gap between thought and reaction, fostering a sense of inner calm and clarity. It also enhances focus, reduces stress, and strengthens the connection between mind and body. Over time, meditation helps dissolve the barriers of ego, revealing a deeper state of consciousness that transcends ordinary perception.

Creative visualization and meditation are often accompanied by the practice of gratitude. Gratitude shifts the mind's focus from what is lacking to what is abundant, fostering a sense of fulfillment and peace. Neuroscience has shown that gratitude activates the brain's reward centers, releasing dopamine and serotonin—chemicals associated with happiness. By cultivating a daily gratitude practice, such as writing down three things one is thankful for, individuals reframe their perspectives and create a foundation of positivity.

The mind's influence extends beyond the individual, radiating outward to affect relationships and the environment. Studies on collective consciousness suggest that when groups meditate or focus their thoughts on peace, crime rates and conflict in surrounding areas decrease. This phenomenon, often called the Maharishi Effect, demonstrates the interconnectedness of minds and the potential for collective transformation.

Another fascinating aspect of mental power is its role in physical healing. The placebo effect, where patients experience real improvements in health despite receiving inactive treatments, highlights the profound connection between belief and biology. This mind-body link is further demonstrated in practices like biofeedback, where individuals learn to control physiological processes such as heart rate and blood pressure through mental focus.

In the realm of personal growth, the mind is both a mirror and a guide. It reflects inner truths and offers insights into one's beliefs, fears, and desires. Journaling, for instance, allows individuals to articulate and process their thoughts, uncovering patterns that may be holding them back. By engaging with the mind in this way, people can clarify their intentions and align their actions with their values.

The mind also holds the key to unlocking intuition. While intuition is often associated with the heart or gut, it is deeply connected to the mind's ability to synthesize information from subtle cues and subconscious knowledge. By quieting the mental chatter through practices like meditation, individuals can access this inner wisdom and make decisions with greater clarity and confidence.

Yet, with all its potential, the mind can also be a source of limitation. Fear, doubt, and negative self-talk can create barriers that prevent individuals from realizing their full potential. Overcoming these obstacles requires not only awareness but also deliberate action. Techniques such as cognitive behavioral therapy (CBT) help individuals identify and challenge distorted thinking patterns, replacing them with balanced and realistic perspectives.

The relationship between the mind and emotions is another critical area of exploration. Thoughts and feelings are deeply intertwined, each influencing the other in a continuous feedback loop. By shifting mental focus, individuals can alter their emotional states, transforming anxiety into calm or frustration into compassion. Practices like emotional regulation and mindfulness-based stress reduction (MBSR) provide tools for navigating this interplay with grace and resilience.

Beyond the individual, the mind plays a pivotal role in shaping societal and cultural narratives. Beliefs, biases, and collective ideologies are all products of shared mental constructs. Recognizing this, the holistic individual seeks to question inherited paradigms and cultivate a mindset of inclusivity and growth. By challenging limiting societal norms and embracing diversity, they contribute to a more conscious and equitable world.

The power of the mind is not confined to intellect or logic; it encompasses imagination, emotion, and spirit. It is the bridge between the tangible and the intangible, the conscious and the unconscious. Through practices that nurture mental clarity, creativity, and awareness, individuals can tap into the limitless potential of this remarkable tool.

The journey of mastering the mind is ongoing, requiring patience, discipline, and self-compassion. Yet, each step brings profound rewards—a deeper sense of self-awareness, a greater capacity for joy, and an expanded ability to manifest one's highest aspirations. By harnessing the power of the mind, individuals not only transform their own lives but also contribute to the collective evolution of humanity.

In the end, the mind is more than an instrument; it is a gateway to the infinite. By learning to navigate its landscapes with intention and wisdom, the holistic individual discovers that the true power of the mind lies not in control, but in alignment— with oneself, with others, and with the universal flow of life.

Chapter 8
Conscious Relationships

Human connection is one of the most profound experiences of existence. Relationships, whether romantic, familial, or platonic, shape our emotions, inform our beliefs, and influence our personal growth. Conscious relationships transcend superficial interactions, embracing authenticity, empathy, and intentionality. They are partnerships rooted in mutual respect and shared growth, offering a space for both individuals to flourish while navigating the challenges and joys of human connection.

The foundation of a conscious relationship begins with self-awareness. To connect deeply with another, one must first cultivate an understanding of their own needs, values, and emotions. This inner work reveals patterns, often rooted in childhood experiences, that influence how we relate to others. By recognizing and addressing these patterns, individuals can break free from reactive behaviors and enter relationships with greater clarity and intention.

Authenticity is the cornerstone of conscious relationships. It requires the courage to show up as one's true self, without masks or pretenses. This vulnerability fosters trust, creating a safe space where both partners can express their feelings and thoughts without fear of judgment. Authenticity does not mean perfection; it means embracing one's flaws and allowing others to see them. In doing so, relationships become genuine and deeply fulfilling.

Empathy is another essential element. Conscious relationships thrive on the ability to step into another's perspective, to feel their emotions and understand their experiences. Empathy builds bridges where differences might otherwise create division. It is the practice of listening not just to respond, but to truly hear and validate the other person's feelings. This act of presence fosters a sense of connection that transcends words.

Communication is the lifeblood of any relationship, and in conscious partnerships, it takes on a deeper significance. Clear, honest, and compassionate communication prevents misunderstandings and resolves conflicts. Techniques such as nonviolent communication (NVC) guide individuals to express their needs and desires without blame or criticism. For example, instead of saying, "You never listen to me," a more conscious approach would be, "I feel unheard when our conversations are interrupted." This shifts the focus from accusation to connection.

Boundaries are another critical aspect of conscious relationships. Setting boundaries is an act of self-love, ensuring that one's emotional and mental well-being is protected. It is not about creating walls but about establishing guidelines for respectful interaction. In healthy relationships, boundaries are mutually respected and viewed as tools for strengthening the partnership.

Conflict, inevitable in any relationship, is viewed differently in a conscious context. Rather than seeing it as a threat, it is embraced as an opportunity for growth and understanding. Conflicts often arise from unmet needs or misaligned expectations, and addressing them requires patience and curiosity. Conscious partners approach disagreements with the intention to learn, asking questions like, "What is this situation teaching us?" or "How can we grow stronger through this challenge?"

Conscious relationships also prioritize quality time and intentional presence. In the fast-paced modern world, it is easy to fall into the habit of superficial interactions. However, conscious connections are nurtured through deep conversations, shared experiences, and undivided attention. Whether it's a quiet evening together or a heartfelt conversation, these moments strengthen the bond and reaffirm the partnership's purpose.

Romantic relationships within the conscious framework move beyond traditional dynamics. They are not solely about companionship or physical attraction but about spiritual alignment and mutual evolution. These partnerships serve as mirrors, reflecting one's strengths and areas for growth. When approached with mindfulness, romantic relationships become sacred spaces for healing, creativity, and transformation.

In familial relationships, the conscious approach seeks to honor both individuality and unity. Parents, for example, cultivate conscious relationships with their children by encouraging open dialogue, modeling emotional intelligence, and respecting their child's unique journey. This creates a foundation of trust and love that supports the child's growth into a confident and authentic individual.

Friendships also benefit from the principles of conscious connection. True friendships are characterized by mutual support, honesty, and shared values. They are spaces where individuals can celebrate each other's successes, offer comfort during challenges, and inspire one another to reach their potential. A conscious friendship is not about frequency of contact but depth of connection, where even time apart does not weaken the bond.

One of the most transformative aspects of conscious relationships is their ability to foster personal growth. Through connection with others, individuals learn patience, compassion, and resilience. Relationships challenge individuals to confront their shadows—the insecurities, fears, and wounds that often lie hidden. By navigating these challenges together, partners create a space for healing and growth that benefits both individuals and the relationship as a whole.

Conscious relationships are also deeply intertwined with spirituality. They recognize that love is not merely an emotion but an energetic force that transcends the physical realm. By fostering love within a relationship, individuals contribute to the collective energy of the world. Acts of kindness, forgiveness, and understanding ripple outward, creating a positive impact far beyond the immediate partnership.

Rituals can play a significant role in cultivating conscious relationships. Simple practices like expressing daily gratitude, sharing affirmations, or meditating together deepen the connection. For example, partners might set aside time each week to reflect on their relationship, discussing what they appreciate about each other and what areas could use more attention. These rituals create a sense of intention and continuity, reinforcing the bond.

The journey toward conscious relationships is not without challenges. It requires a willingness to confront uncomfortable truths, embrace vulnerability, and let go of ego-driven behaviors. However, the rewards—deeper intimacy, mutual respect, and authentic connection—make the effort worthwhile.

One inspiring example of conscious connection is seen in long-term partnerships that continue to evolve over decades. These relationships thrive not because they are free of conflict, but because both individuals are committed to growth and alignment. They view their partnership as a dynamic entity, one that requires nurturing, reflection, and adaptability.

Similarly, conscious relationships extend to the broader community. Acts of kindness toward strangers, collaboration within teams, and support for collective causes all reflect the principles of empathy and intentionality. These connections remind us that every relationship, no matter how fleeting, holds the potential for meaningful impact.

Ultimately, conscious relationships teach us that love is not a possession but a practice. It is not about finding the perfect partner or avoiding conflict but about showing up with presence, authenticity, and compassion. Through these relationships, we discover the beauty of human connection and the transformative power of love.

As individuals embark on the path of conscious relationships, they learn to see others not as separate but as reflections of themselves. This shift in perspective fosters unity, dissolving barriers and creating a world where connection is celebrated as the foundation of life. Through conscious relationships, we learn not only how to love others but also how to love ourselves, and in doing so, we contribute to a more harmonious and compassionate world.

Chapter 9
Purposeful Work

Work, at its core, is more than a means of survival; it is a channel through which we express our creativity, contribute to society, and align with our purpose. For the holistic individual, purposeful work is not just about financial gain or external recognition—it is about finding fulfillment and harmony between one's talents, passions, and values. It is a journey toward aligning daily efforts with a deeper sense of meaning, creating a life that feels both productive and intentional.

Purposeful work begins with self-discovery. Before one can align their career with their inner calling, it is essential to understand their strengths, interests, and motivations. This process often involves introspection and asking profound questions: What brings me joy? What challenges inspire me to grow? How can my work serve others while remaining true to my values? The answers to these questions provide a foundation for identifying a vocation that resonates with the soul.

For some, the search for purpose reveals a need to shift careers entirely, moving toward roles that reflect their authentic desires. Others may find that purposeful work does not require a change in occupation but rather a change in perspective—infusing their current role with more intention, creativity, and connection. A teacher, for example, may rediscover their purpose by viewing their role as not merely imparting knowledge but shaping the lives of future generations.

Entrepreneurship often becomes a path for those seeking purposeful work. Creating a business or venture aligned with one's values offers the freedom to innovate and express individuality. Holistic entrepreneurs frequently pursue fields such as wellness, sustainability, and education, where their efforts can make a positive impact on others and the planet. These ventures are often guided by principles such as conscious capitalism, which prioritizes ethical practices, environmental stewardship, and community well-being over short-term profit.

One of the hallmarks of purposeful work is the integration of personal values into professional life. This alignment transforms work from a source of stress into a source of inspiration. For instance, someone passionate about environmental sustainability may find purpose in working for a green energy company or leading initiatives to reduce waste in their organization. Similarly, individuals with a strong sense of empathy might thrive in roles within healthcare, counseling, or social advocacy, where their compassion becomes a driving force for positive change.

Balance is another key aspect of purposeful work. Holistic individuals recognize that while work is an important part of life, it is not the entirety of it. Burnout and overwork often stem from a misalignment between personal well-being and professional demands. Purposeful work seeks to create harmony, ensuring that time for rest, relationships, and self-care is valued alongside productivity. Practices such as setting boundaries, prioritizing tasks, and adopting mindfulness at work help maintain this equilibrium.

The concept of a "soul-aligned career" has gained prominence in the modern holistic movement. This approach views work as an extension of one's spiritual path, where each task becomes an opportunity for growth and expression. Whether it is crafting a product, solving a complex problem, or leading a team, purposeful work transforms mundane responsibilities into acts of service and creativity. It encourages individuals to bring their whole selves to their work, merging professional skill with personal integrity.

Mindfulness practices are invaluable in creating a sense of purpose in the workplace. By cultivating presence and awareness, individuals can approach their tasks with greater focus and intention. A simple mindfulness exercise, such as taking a few deep breaths before starting a project, shifts the energy from stress to clarity. Over time, this practice fosters a deeper connection to the work itself, making even routine tasks feel meaningful.

Collaboration is another hallmark of purposeful work. Holistic individuals view their colleagues not as competitors but as partners in a shared mission. This perspective fosters an environment of mutual respect, open communication, and collective creativity. Teams that operate with a sense of shared purpose are often more innovative, resilient, and harmonious, as each member feels valued and aligned with the group's goals.

Leadership takes on a transformative dimension in the context of purposeful work. Holistic leaders inspire by example, demonstrating empathy, integrity, and vision. They prioritize the well-being of their teams, creating environments where individuals feel empowered to contribute their best. These leaders recognize that success is not solely measured by profits or accolades but by the positive impact their work has on people and the planet.

Purposeful work also embraces the concept of "right livelihood," a term from Buddhist teachings that emphasizes ethical and mindful approaches to earning a living. Right livelihood encourages individuals to choose professions that do not harm others or the environment, promoting activities that contribute to collective well-being. This principle serves as a guide for those seeking to align their careers with their values, reminding them that true success is measured by the positive difference they make in the world.

For those in creative professions, purposeful work often means channeling their artistic talents into projects that inspire and uplift. Writers, musicians, and artists can infuse their work with themes of hope, resilience, and connection, using their craft as a medium for storytelling and transformation. By sharing their authentic voices, they contribute to the collective human experience, reminding others of the beauty and meaning in life.

Purposeful work does not always involve grand gestures or high-profile careers. Small, everyday acts of service and dedication are equally powerful. A barista who greets customers with genuine warmth, a janitor who takes pride in maintaining a clean and welcoming space, or a volunteer who dedicates their time to a local cause—all embody the spirit of purposeful work. It is not the role itself but the intention and presence brought to it that creates meaning.

The journey to discovering purposeful work is often nonlinear. It may involve moments of doubt, trial, and error. However, each step along the way provides valuable insights, helping individuals refine their understanding of what truly matters to them. Patience and openness are essential, as the path to purpose often unfolds in unexpected ways.

One inspiring example of purposeful work is the rise of social enterprises—businesses that prioritize social and environmental goals alongside financial sustainability. These ventures address pressing global issues, from poverty to climate change, demonstrating that work can be both impactful and fulfilling. Whether it's a company that provides clean water to underserved communities or an organization that empowers marginalized groups, these enterprises embody the principles of holistic purpose.

Another example is the growing movement toward remote and flexible work. By allowing individuals to design their schedules around their personal rhythms and needs, these arrangements create opportunities for greater balance and fulfillment. For many, working from home or choosing freelance opportunities has opened the door to pursuing passion projects and cultivating deeper connections with family and community.

Purposeful work also inspires individuals to think beyond themselves. It encourages contributions to a greater cause, whether through mentorship, volunteering, or advocacy. These acts of service remind us that our work has the power to ripple outward, touching lives and creating positive change far beyond our immediate circle.

In embracing purposeful work, individuals reconnect with their innate creativity and drive. They transform challenges into opportunities for growth and redefine success as living in alignment with their values. Purposeful work is not just a career choice; it is a way of being, where every action becomes a reflection of one's highest intentions.

Ultimately, purposeful work is about more than what we do; it is about how and why we do it. It is an invitation to approach life with curiosity, courage, and commitment, creating a legacy that reflects our deepest truths. Through purposeful work, we discover not only what we are capable of achieving but also the profound joy of contributing to something greater than ourselves.

Chapter 10
Meditation and Silence

In the chaotic noise of modern life, where distractions pull at every corner of the mind, the practice of meditation and silence emerges as a sanctuary. These ancient tools, rooted in timeless traditions, offer a path to inner peace, clarity, and connection. Meditation and silence are more than just practices; they are gateways to the self, spaces where the mind quiets, and the soul speaks.

At its essence, meditation is the art of presence. It is the practice of becoming fully aware of the moment, observing thoughts without attachment, and grounding oneself in the now. While its origins span diverse spiritual traditions—from the meditative chants of Hinduism to the contemplative prayers of Christianity—meditation transcends religious boundaries, offering universal benefits to those who seek stillness and insight.

Silence, often overlooked in its profound simplicity, complements meditation as a powerful tool for self-discovery. In silence, the external distractions fade away, revealing the subtleties of thought, emotion, and intuition. It is in these quiet moments that individuals can hear the whispers of their inner truth, reconnecting with their authentic selves.

The benefits of meditation extend far beyond relaxation. On a physical level, meditation reduces stress by lowering cortisol levels, enhances immune function, and improves heart health. Mentally, it sharpens focus, fosters creativity, and cultivates resilience. Emotionally, it provides a space to process feelings, releasing fear, anger, and sadness while nurturing compassion and joy. Spiritually, meditation aligns the practitioner with a sense of unity, dissolving the boundaries between self and the universe.

There are countless forms of meditation, each offering unique pathways to stillness and awareness. Mindfulness meditation, rooted in Buddhist traditions, emphasizes observing the breath, bodily sensations, and thoughts without judgment. This practice grounds individuals in the present moment, allowing them to experience life fully without being consumed by the past or future.

Loving-kindness meditation, or *metta*, cultivates compassion and empathy by directing thoughts of goodwill toward oneself, loved ones, and even those with whom one feels conflict. The repetition of phrases like "May I be happy. May I be healthy. May I live with ease," creates an expansive sense of love that radiates outward.

Transcendental Meditation (TM), popularized in the West, involves silently repeating a mantra—a word or phrase chosen for its vibrational quality. This repetition quiets the mind, creating a state of deep relaxation and heightened awareness. TM is known for its accessibility, requiring minimal effort while yielding profound results.

Guided meditations, often led by teachers or audio recordings, use visualization and narration to help individuals relax, focus, or achieve specific intentions. For example, a guided meditation might lead participants through a serene forest, encouraging them to imagine the sounds, smells, and sensations of nature, fostering a sense of calm and grounding.

Silent meditation retreats, such as Vipassana, take the practice to a deeper level by immersing participants in days or weeks of uninterrupted silence. These retreats strip away external distractions, creating a space for profound self-reflection and inner growth. While challenging, the rewards are transformative, often leading to heightened clarity, emotional healing, and spiritual awakening.

The role of breath in meditation cannot be overstated. The breath serves as an anchor, a rhythmic pulse that connects body and mind. Techniques such as *pranayama* (yogic breath control) deepen the meditative experience by regulating the flow of energy within the body. Practices like alternate nostril breathing balance the nervous system, while diaphragmatic breathing promotes relaxation and focus.

Silence, when practiced intentionally, becomes a meditation in itself. Whether through silent walks in nature, periods of quiet solitude, or simply pausing to listen to the world without speaking, silence offers a profound opportunity to connect with the present moment. It allows the mind to settle, revealing insights that are often drowned out by the noise of daily life.

Incorporating meditation and silence into a busy life may seem daunting, but even small practices can create meaningful change. A few minutes of focused breathing in the morning can set a calm tone for the day. Pausing for a moment of stillness before meals cultivates gratitude. Taking a short break to sit in silence during a hectic day restores energy and clarity.

Modern technology, often blamed for fostering distraction, can also support meditative practices. Apps like Headspace, Calm, and Insight Timer provide guided meditations, timers, and reminders to create consistent habits. While technology should not replace the essence of the practice, it can serve as a bridge for beginners or those seeking structure.

Meditation and silence are also tools for navigating life's challenges. During moments of stress, returning to the breath grounds the individual, preventing reactive decision-making. In periods of grief or loss, silence offers a space to process emotions without judgment. When faced with uncertainty, meditation provides clarity and a sense of inner strength.

Stories of transformation through meditation abound. A woman battling anxiety finds solace in mindfulness, learning to observe her thoughts without fear. A man recovering from burnout discovers the power of silence, using it to reconnect with his purpose. Communities that meditate together, such as in schools or workplaces, report increased harmony, focus, and mutual respect.

Meditation also serves as a gateway to deeper spiritual practices. For those on a spiritual path, it becomes a form of prayer or communion with the divine. It is in these quiet moments that individuals often experience profound insights, feelings of oneness, or a connection to something greater than themselves.

Children, too, can benefit from meditation and silence. Teaching mindfulness in schools has shown to improve focus, emotional regulation, and empathy among students. Simple practices, like guiding children to notice their breath or reflect on what they are grateful for, create a foundation of inner peace that they carry into adulthood.

While the benefits of meditation and silence are vast, the journey is not without its challenges. The mind, accustomed to constant stimulation, often resists stillness. Thoughts arise, distractions intrude, and the silence can feel uncomfortable. However, these challenges are part of the process. Meditation is not about achieving a perfect state but about returning to the practice, again and again, with patience and compassion.

For the holistic individual, meditation and silence are more than tools; they are ways of being. They cultivate a life of presence, where each moment is experienced fully, and each action is imbued with intention. They remind us that beneath the noise and chaos of the world lies a stillness that is always accessible—a sanctuary within.

Through meditation and silence, we learn to listen—not just to the external world, but to the depths of our own being. We discover that the answers we seek are often already within us, waiting to be heard. In this stillness, we find clarity, connection, and the profound realization that we are part of a greater whole.

In the embrace of meditation and silence, life slows, the mind settles, and the soul awakens. It is here, in this quiet space, that the true essence of existence reveals itself, reminding us of the beauty and simplicity of simply being.

Chapter 11
Holistic Education

Education, at its most profound, is a journey of self-discovery and empowerment. Holistic education moves beyond conventional academics to address the emotional, creative, and spiritual dimensions of an individual. It is an approach that nurtures the whole person, fostering curiosity, compassion, and a sense of purpose. As traditional models of education evolve, the holistic perspective is gaining traction, offering a transformative framework for lifelong learning.

The principles of holistic education are rooted in interconnectedness. It views each learner as a unique being whose intellectual, emotional, and spiritual growth are inseparable. Rather than focusing solely on standardized outcomes, holistic education prioritizes personal development, creativity, and the cultivation of values such as empathy and resilience.

One of the key aspects of holistic education is emotional learning. Traditional systems often overlook the role of emotions in shaping behavior and decision-making. Holistic education seeks to change this by teaching students how to recognize, process, and express their emotions constructively. Practices like journaling, group discussions, and mindfulness exercises help learners develop emotional intelligence, enabling them to navigate life with confidence and compassion.

Creativity also lies at the heart of holistic education. By encouraging exploration and experimentation, this approach helps students discover their unique talents and passions. Artistic endeavors such as painting, music, and theater are not treated as extracurricular activities but as essential components of learning.

Creativity is seen as a vital skill that fosters innovation, critical thinking, and the ability to approach challenges from multiple perspectives.

Spiritual development, often misunderstood in the context of education, is another vital element. In holistic education, spirituality does not refer to religion but to a sense of connection—whether to oneself, others, or the natural world. This dimension is nurtured through practices like meditation, gratitude, and reflection, which help students cultivate inner peace and purpose.

Experiential learning is a hallmark of holistic education. Instead of relying solely on textbooks and lectures, students are immersed in hands-on experiences that bring concepts to life. For instance, a science lesson might involve gardening to study plant biology, while a history class could include visits to local heritage sites. These experiences make learning tangible, engaging multiple senses and fostering a deeper understanding of the material.

Community plays a significant role in holistic education. Learning is not confined to classrooms but extends into families, neighborhoods, and the broader world. Students are encouraged to collaborate, share knowledge, and contribute to their communities. Projects such as environmental clean-ups, intergenerational storytelling, and service-learning initiatives instill a sense of responsibility and interconnectedness.

The role of teachers in holistic education is transformative. Rather than acting as authoritarian figures, they become mentors and guides, creating a supportive environment where students feel valued and inspired. Holistic educators model empathy, patience, and authenticity, fostering relationships built on trust and mutual respect.

Nature is another integral element of holistic education. Spending time outdoors not only enhances physical health but also nurtures a sense of wonder and connection to the natural world. Activities like forest schools, gardening programs, and nature walks teach students about sustainability, biodiversity, and their role in preserving the planet.

Holistic education also addresses the importance of mindfulness and meditation in the learning process. By teaching students to focus their attention and regulate their emotions, these practices enhance concentration, reduce stress, and improve overall well-being. A simple mindfulness exercise, such as observing the breath for a few moments before a lesson, can create a calm and focused learning environment.

As the world becomes more interconnected and complex, holistic education prepares learners to thrive in diverse and rapidly changing environments. It emphasizes adaptability, collaboration, and the ability to see connections between seemingly unrelated ideas. These skills are essential for addressing global challenges, from climate change to social inequality.

Critics of holistic education often argue that it lacks the rigor of traditional approaches. However, this perspective overlooks the depth and breadth of holistic learning. By addressing multiple dimensions of development, holistic education produces well-rounded individuals who are not only academically capable but also emotionally intelligent, creatively inspired, and socially conscious.

Examples of holistic education in action can be found worldwide. In Finland, one of the most progressive education systems, schools emphasize play, creativity, and student-led learning. Montessori schools, founded on principles of self-directed exploration, encourage students to follow their interests while developing independence and responsibility. Waldorf education, another holistic model, integrates academics, arts, and practical skills to nurture balanced growth.

Technology, when used mindfully, can enhance holistic education. Digital tools such as virtual reality, online collaboration platforms, and educational apps provide new ways to explore and connect. However, holistic educators caution against over-reliance on screens, emphasizing the importance of face-to-face interaction and hands-on activities.

Parents and caregivers also play a crucial role in supporting holistic education. By fostering a home environment that values curiosity, empathy, and open communication, they complement the efforts of teachers and schools. Simple practices like reading together, discussing current events, or exploring hobbies as a family create opportunities for shared learning and connection.

Holistic education is not limited to children; it is a lifelong journey. Adults can embrace its principles through personal development courses, mindfulness workshops, and community engagement. By committing to continuous growth, individuals contribute to a culture of learning that transcends age and background.

The ultimate goal of holistic education is not merely to produce successful individuals but to nurture compassionate, creative, and conscious global citizens. It is about empowering learners to lead lives of purpose and integrity, contributing to a world that values connection, balance, and sustainability.

In the rapidly evolving landscape of the 21st century, holistic education offers a beacon of hope. It reminds us that true learning is not just about acquiring knowledge but about cultivating wisdom, empathy, and the courage to make a difference. Through this approach, education becomes not just a means to an end but a transformative journey that enriches every aspect of life.

Chapter 12
The Inner Universe

The journey toward self-discovery is one of the most profound paths a person can take. Within each of us lies an intricate and vast inner universe, a realm of thoughts, emotions, beliefs, and untapped potential. Exploring this inner world allows us to uncover the truths that define us, the patterns that shape us, and the purpose that drives us. This chapter delves into the depths of self-awareness, guiding the reader through the process of navigating their inner landscape to cultivate a life of authenticity and fulfillment.

At the heart of the inner universe is the concept of self-awareness. To know oneself is to understand the layers that make up who we are—our strengths, fears, desires, and limitations. Self-awareness begins with observation, the act of stepping back from the constant chatter of the mind to notice what lies beneath. This practice is not about judgment but about curiosity, a gentle inquiry into the habits, reactions, and emotions that govern our lives.

One of the most transformative tools for exploring the inner universe is introspection. This practice invites us to ask questions that reveal the deeper truths of our existence. Why do we react the way we do? What beliefs do we hold about ourselves and the world? How do these beliefs shape our reality? Through introspection, we uncover the narratives that have been unconsciously guiding us, allowing us to rewrite the stories that no longer serve us.

Central to this exploration is the recognition of limiting beliefs. These are the internalized thoughts and assumptions that create barriers to growth and fulfillment. Often formed during childhood, limiting beliefs might include ideas like "I'm not good enough," "Success is unattainable," or "I don't deserve love." While these beliefs may feel like truths, they are simply mental constructs that can be dismantled with awareness and intention.

To address limiting beliefs, it is essential to replace them with empowering ones. Affirmations, visualization, and self-compassion practices can help reframe negative thought patterns. For example, replacing "I'm not capable" with "I am capable of learning and growing" shifts the mindset from limitation to possibility. Over time, these new beliefs become the foundation for confidence and resilience.

Emotions are another vital aspect of the inner universe. Each emotion, whether joy or sadness, anger or gratitude, is a messenger offering insight into our needs and values. Emotional awareness requires us to sit with our feelings, to name them without judgment, and to understand their origins. Practices like journaling and mindful reflection create a safe space to process emotions, transforming them from sources of pain into pathways for healing.

The concept of shadow work plays a pivotal role in navigating the inner universe. The shadow, as described by psychologist Carl Jung, represents the parts of ourselves that we suppress or deny—our fears, insecurities, and unhealed wounds. While the shadow may seem intimidating, it is also a source of immense power and growth. By facing our shadow with courage and compassion, we integrate these hidden aspects into our consciousness, becoming more whole and authentic.

Meditation is a powerful ally in exploring the inner universe. By quieting the mind, meditation creates a space to observe thoughts and emotions without attachment. Over time, this practice deepens self-awareness, revealing the patterns and insights that lie beneath the surface. Techniques like body scans, loving-kindness meditations, and mindfulness practices help cultivate a greater connection to oneself.

Another tool for self-discovery is the practice of asking reflective questions. These questions, when explored with honesty, guide us toward clarity and alignment. For example:

- What truly matters to me?
- What am I holding onto that no longer serves me?
- How do I want to contribute to the world?

These inquiries act as signposts on the journey through the inner universe, leading us closer to our authentic selves.

Creativity also plays a key role in this journey. Artistic expression—whether through painting, writing, music, or dance—offers a way to access and explore the subconscious mind. These creative outlets provide a channel for emotions and insights that words alone cannot express. They allow us to connect with the intuitive, non-linear aspects of our being, uncovering wisdom that often lies beyond logic.

Self-compassion is essential when navigating the inner universe. The process of self-discovery can bring up painful memories or uncomfortable truths. Meeting these experiences with kindness and understanding creates a nurturing environment for growth. Self-compassion reminds us that we are not defined by our mistakes or flaws but by our willingness to learn and evolve.

The inner universe also holds the key to our passions and purpose. By tuning into what excites and inspires us, we align with the activities and goals that bring meaning to our lives. This alignment creates a sense of flow, where our actions feel natural and fulfilling. Discovering our purpose is not about finding a single answer but about living in a way that reflects our values and gifts.

As we explore the inner universe, we begin to see the connections between our inner world and the external one. Our thoughts influence our actions, our emotions shape our relationships, and our beliefs create the lens through which we view life. This interconnectedness reminds us that the work we do within ourselves ripples outward, affecting every aspect of our existence.

Navigating the inner universe is not a linear journey but a lifelong process. There will be moments of clarity and moments of confusion, periods of growth and times of rest. The key is to approach the journey with patience, curiosity, and an open heart.

Stories of transformation illustrate the power of this journey. A man burdened by self-doubt begins journaling, uncovering the beliefs that have held him back. Through reflection and mindfulness, he learns to embrace his strengths and pursue his dreams. A woman recovering from trauma uses meditation and shadow work to process her pain, emerging with a deeper sense of resilience and self-love.

The beauty of the inner universe is its infinite depth. No matter how much we explore, there is always more to discover, more to heal, and more to celebrate. It is a realm of endless potential, a testament to the complexity and richness of the human experience.

Ultimately, the journey through the inner universe leads to greater authenticity, peace, and empowerment. It teaches us that we are not defined by external circumstances but by the choices we make and the love we cultivate within ourselves. Through this journey, we come to understand that the greatest adventure lies not in seeking what is outside but in discovering the boundless possibilities within.

Chapter 13
The Energy of Love

Love is the most transformative energy in the universe, a force that transcends boundaries and connects all living beings. It is not merely an emotion or a fleeting feeling; love is an energetic state that permeates every aspect of existence. When embraced holistically, love becomes a powerful tool for healing, growth, and connection—both within ourselves and with the world around us.

At its core, the energy of love is unconditional. It does not judge, demand, or expect; it simply flows, uniting and elevating. Love begins with self, radiates outward to others, and ultimately connects us to the greater whole. This energy is accessible to everyone, yet truly embodying it requires intentional practice and an open heart.

Self-love is the foundation of the energy of love. Without a deep sense of acceptance and compassion for ourselves, it is difficult to fully love others. Self-love is not selfish or indulgent—it is the recognition of our inherent worth and the willingness to care for ourselves as we would a beloved friend. Practices like positive affirmations, self-care rituals, and setting healthy boundaries cultivate this essential relationship with oneself.

The energy of love also thrives in relationships. When we approach others with empathy, understanding, and authenticity, we create spaces where love can flourish. Conscious relationships, as explored earlier, are built on this energetic foundation. They prioritize listening, mutual respect, and the willingness to grow together. Through love, conflicts transform into opportunities for deeper connection, and challenges become shared journeys.

Forgiveness is one of the most potent expressions of the energy of love. Holding onto resentment or anger keeps us bound to pain, whereas forgiveness liberates us. It is not about condoning harmful actions but about releasing their grip on our hearts. Forgiveness is an act of love that heals both the giver and the receiver, restoring harmony to relationships and inner peace to the soul.

Love also manifests as service to others. Acts of kindness, generosity, and compassion are tangible expressions of this energy. Whether helping a neighbor, volunteering in the community, or simply offering a smile to a stranger, these actions create ripples of positivity. They remind us that love is not limited to grand gestures but is present in the smallest, most heartfelt moments.

Energetically, love operates at a high frequency. When we embody love, we raise our vibration, which influences our health, emotions, and interactions. Scientific studies support this connection; emotions like gratitude and love have been shown to positively affect the heart's rhythm, promoting coherence and resilience. Conversely, states like fear and anger create chaotic energy patterns that disrupt balance.

Practices like heart-centered meditation enhance the energy of love. By focusing attention on the heart and visualizing it radiating light, we can amplify feelings of love and compassion. This practice not only uplifts our mood but also strengthens our energetic field, making us more receptive to love and more capable of sharing it with others.

The energy of love extends beyond personal relationships to include a connection with the universe itself. Many spiritual traditions view love as the essence of the divine, a unifying force that flows through all creation. By aligning with this energy, we tap into a sense of oneness, recognizing that we are interconnected with every living being and the cosmos.

Gratitude is another powerful pathway to the energy of love. When we focus on what we appreciate, we shift our perspective from lack to abundance. Gratitude deepens our awareness of the love present in our lives, from the support of friends and family to the beauty of nature. Keeping a gratitude journal or reflecting on moments of joy helps anchor this energy, fostering a mindset of love and appreciation.

Love is also a catalyst for personal transformation. It encourages us to confront our fears, embrace vulnerability, and transcend limitations. The energy of love dissolves the barriers we build around our hearts, allowing us to connect more deeply with ourselves and others. In this way, love is both the journey and the destination—a force that guides us toward our highest potential.

Healing is one of the most profound aspects of love's energy. Whether physical, emotional, or spiritual, love has the power to mend what is broken. Studies on the placebo effect, for example, demonstrate how belief and care—both forms of love—can accelerate healing. Similarly, practices like Reiki and energy work channel love to restore balance and vitality.

In a broader sense, the energy of love is essential for the well-being of the planet. Environmental stewardship, social justice, and community building are all acts of love on a collective scale. When we care for the earth and its inhabitants, we align with the holistic principle that love is not confined to individuals but extends to all of existence.

Love also teaches us about acceptance. To love unconditionally is to embrace life as it is, without trying to control or change it. This does not mean resigning ourselves to harmful situations but rather approaching challenges with an open heart and a willingness to learn. Acceptance allows us to flow with the rhythms of life, finding peace in the midst of uncertainty.

The energy of love is often most evident in times of adversity. During crises, people come together to support one another, demonstrating the strength and resilience of love. These moments remind us that love is not diminished by hardship but grows stronger through acts of courage and compassion.

While love is universal, the ways we express it are deeply personal. Some show love through words of affirmation, others through acts of service or physical touch. Understanding these different expressions, often referred to as "love languages," helps us communicate love more effectively. It also deepens our appreciation for the unique ways others share their hearts.

One of the greatest lessons of love is that it is not finite. The more we give, the more we receive. Love is a self-renewing resource, a wellspring that grows as we draw from it. By sharing love freely, we create a cycle of abundance that enriches everyone it touches.

Ultimately, the energy of love is the essence of what it means to be human. It is the thread that connects us to one another, to the earth, and to the universe. Through love, we find purpose, healing, and joy. It is a force that transforms not only individuals but the world, reminding us that we are all part of something greater than ourselves.

In embracing the energy of love, we align with the highest vibrations of existence. We learn to see beauty in the ordinary, to find connection in diversity, and to approach life with an open and generous heart. Love, in its purest form, is the most powerful energy we possess—a guiding light that illuminates the path to wholeness and harmony.

Chapter 14
Holism in Technology

In a world increasingly shaped by rapid technological advancements, the relationship between technology and holistic living may seem paradoxical. Technology is often associated with disconnection, overstimulation, and the erosion of natural rhythms. However, when approached mindfully, technology has the potential to become a powerful ally in the holistic journey, serving as a tool for growth, connection, and balance. This chapter explores how technology can be integrated into a holistic lifestyle, emphasizing its role as a means to enhance well-being rather than detract from it.

At its core, the holistic approach to technology begins with intentionality. Rather than allowing devices and platforms to dictate our time and attention, we must consciously choose how to engage with them. This means using technology as a tool to support our values and goals, rather than as a source of distraction or dependency. The first step in this process is cultivating awareness of how technology affects our physical, mental, and emotional states.

One of the most transformative ways technology can support holistic living is through mindfulness and meditation apps. Platforms such as Headspace, Calm, and Insight Timer offer guided meditations, breathing exercises, and sleep aids designed to help users manage stress, improve focus, and cultivate inner peace. These tools make ancient practices accessible to modern audiences, allowing individuals to integrate mindfulness into their daily routines with ease.

Wearable technology also plays a significant role in promoting health and balance. Devices like fitness trackers and smartwatches monitor physical activity, heart rate, sleep patterns, and even stress levels, providing valuable insights into one's overall well-being. By using this data, individuals can make informed decisions about their health, creating personalized routines that align with their unique needs.

Technology's potential for connection is another key aspect of its integration into holistic living. Social media, when used mindfully, allows people to share ideas, find support, and build communities around shared interests. Online platforms dedicated to wellness, spirituality, and sustainability provide spaces for like-minded individuals to connect, collaborate, and inspire one another. Virtual events, workshops, and retreats have made holistic practices more accessible than ever, transcending geographical boundaries and fostering a sense of global unity.

In education, technology enhances holistic learning by offering a wealth of resources on topics such as meditation, nutrition, and energy healing. Online courses, webinars, and digital libraries empower individuals to explore and deepen their understanding of holistic practices at their own pace. Additionally, virtual reality (VR) is emerging as a tool for immersive experiences, allowing users to explore serene natural landscapes, practice yoga, or engage in guided meditations from the comfort of their homes.

Technology also plays a vital role in sustainability, a cornerstone of holistic living. Smart home devices, such as energy-efficient thermostats and lighting systems, reduce energy consumption and promote eco-conscious living. Apps that track carbon footprints, encourage recycling, and suggest sustainable alternatives empower individuals to make environmentally friendly choices. Platforms like Ecosia, a search engine that plants trees with every search, demonstrate how technology can align with holistic values to create positive global impact.

Despite these benefits, it is essential to address the challenges and potential pitfalls of technology. Overuse or misuse of devices can lead to digital fatigue, disrupted sleep patterns, and diminished attention spans. Social media, while a tool for connection, can also foster comparison, anxiety, and isolation if not approached with mindfulness. Recognizing these risks, the holistic individual seeks to establish healthy boundaries with technology, ensuring that its use remains purposeful and balanced.

Digital detoxes, for example, provide an opportunity to disconnect from screens and reconnect with the present moment. Whether for a few hours, a day, or a weekend, stepping away from technology allows individuals to recharge, reflect, and re-establish a sense of inner calm. Simple practices, such as turning off notifications, setting device-free zones, or limiting screen time before bed, create space for more meaningful engagement with oneself and others.

The design of technology itself is also evolving to align with holistic principles. Developers are increasingly focusing on creating tools that prioritize well-being, accessibility, and sustainability. For instance, apps that promote gratitude journaling, digital planners designed for mindful productivity, and platforms that encourage meaningful social interactions reflect a shift toward more conscious design.

One of the most promising frontiers in the integration of technology and holism is artificial intelligence (AI). AI-powered platforms have the potential to revolutionize personalized wellness by analyzing individual needs and offering tailored recommendations for nutrition, exercise, and stress management. While this technology is still developing, its potential to enhance holistic living is vast—provided it is implemented ethically and responsibly.

For businesses and organizations, the holistic approach to technology emphasizes creating environments that support employee well-being. Remote work technologies, wellness apps, and virtual collaboration tools enable flexible work arrangements that prioritize balance and mental health. Forward-thinking companies are also using technology to foster community, offering virtual mindfulness sessions, wellness challenges, and platforms for peer support.

Technology's ability to foster connection extends beyond individuals to include the natural world. Apps like iNaturalist, which help users identify and learn about local flora and fauna, encourage a deeper appreciation for nature. Tools for sustainable agriculture, such as precision farming technologies, support eco-friendly food production and contribute to a healthier planet.

To fully integrate technology into a holistic lifestyle, it is important to approach it with discernment and intention. This means asking questions like:

- Does this tool enhance my well-being or distract from it?
- Is my use of technology aligned with my values and goals?
- How can I create balance in my digital and offline life?

Answering these questions helps individuals cultivate a mindful relationship with technology, ensuring that its benefits are maximized while its drawbacks are minimized.

Stories of transformation illustrate the potential of technology when used holistically. A busy professional finds peace through a daily meditation app, reclaiming moments of calm in a hectic schedule. A family reduces their environmental impact by using smart home devices to monitor energy use. A community of wellness practitioners connects through an online platform, sharing insights and support that enrich their collective journey.

Ultimately, the role of technology in holistic living is not about replacing traditional practices but enhancing them. It is a bridge that connects ancient wisdom with modern innovation, making holistic principles more accessible and applicable in today's world. When approached with mindfulness and intention, technology becomes not a barrier but a partner in the journey toward balance, growth, and connection.

In the end, holism in technology is about integration. It is the recognition that tools, when used consciously, can align with our highest aspirations. By embracing technology as a means to support our values and well-being, we create a harmonious relationship with the digital world—one that enriches our lives and fosters a deeper connection to ourselves, others, and the planet.

Chapter 15
Resilience and Balance

Resilience and balance are the twin pillars that enable holistic individuals to navigate life's inevitable challenges with grace and strength. Resilience is the capacity to recover, adapt, and thrive in the face of adversity, while balance is the state of harmony that sustains well-being across physical, emotional, mental, and spiritual dimensions. Together, they form the foundation for a life lived with intention, peace, and purpose.

In the holistic framework, resilience is not merely about enduring hardships but about growing through them. It is the ability to transform obstacles into opportunities for self-discovery and growth. This perspective shifts the narrative from survival to evolution, encouraging individuals to view challenges as stepping stones toward greater awareness and empowerment.

The first step in cultivating resilience is self-awareness. Understanding one's triggers, strengths, and vulnerabilities allows for a proactive approach to adversity. Journaling, mindfulness, and introspective practices help uncover the patterns that influence reactions to stress, providing insights into how to respond with greater intention.

Mindset plays a crucial role in resilience. A growth mindset—the belief that challenges are opportunities to learn and improve—fosters adaptability and perseverance. By reframing setbacks as lessons rather than failures, individuals develop the confidence and courage to move forward. This mental flexibility transforms obstacles into catalysts for transformation.

Emotional regulation is another cornerstone of resilience. The ability to process and navigate emotions, rather than suppressing or being overwhelmed by them, creates stability in the face of turmoil. Practices such as breathwork, meditation, and emotional release techniques help individuals stay grounded, even during times of uncertainty.

Social connections are vital for building resilience. Supportive relationships provide a sense of belonging, encouragement, and perspective during difficult times. Whether through family, friends, or community networks, cultivating authentic connections creates a safety net that bolsters emotional and mental well-being. Holistic individuals prioritize quality over quantity in their relationships, seeking mutual respect, empathy, and trust.

Balance, the companion of resilience, is about creating harmony across all aspects of life. It involves aligning daily routines, habits, and priorities with one's values and needs. Balance is not about perfection or rigidity but about dynamic equilibrium—a fluid state that adapts to the changing circumstances of life.

Physical balance begins with self-care. Nutrition, movement, and rest form the foundation of a healthy body capable of withstanding stress. Holistic individuals adopt practices that honor their unique needs, whether through yoga, tai chi, mindful eating, or prioritizing restorative sleep. These habits nourish the body and create a stable base from which to face challenges.

Mental balance is cultivated through practices that enhance focus and clarity. Mindfulness, time management, and setting boundaries around work and technology create the mental space needed for creativity and problem-solving. Holistic individuals also embrace the importance of play and curiosity, allowing time for activities that bring joy and inspire exploration.

Emotional balance requires acknowledging and honoring one's feelings without being ruled by them. Gratitude practices, affirmations, and emotional journaling help foster a positive emotional state. By creating rituals to process and release negative emotions, individuals maintain emotional harmony and prevent burnout.

Spiritual balance comes from connecting with something greater than oneself, whether through meditation, nature, or acts of service. This connection provides a sense of purpose and perspective, reminding individuals of their place within the larger tapestry of life. Practices such as gratitude, prayer, or energy work strengthen this bond, anchoring individuals in a sense of trust and flow.

Resilience and balance are also deeply interconnected. A balanced life creates the foundation for resilience, while resilience allows individuals to regain balance after disruptions. Together, they create a cycle of renewal, where each strengthens and reinforces the other.

One of the most effective ways to cultivate resilience and balance is through daily rituals. These small, consistent practices serve as anchors, providing stability and structure amidst the unpredictability of life. For instance, starting the day with a mindfulness meditation sets a calm and intentional tone, while ending the day with a gratitude journal fosters reflection and peace.

Boundaries are another essential tool for maintaining balance. Saying no to excessive demands, creating device-free times, and protecting personal time for rest and reflection ensure that energy is not depleted unnecessarily. Holistic individuals understand that boundaries are not barriers but acts of self-respect that preserve well-being.

Resilience also grows through embracing change. Life is inherently unpredictable, and resistance to change often creates unnecessary suffering. By cultivating acceptance and adaptability, individuals can flow with life's currents rather than struggling against them. Practices like visualization and affirmations help reframe change as an opportunity for growth, fostering a sense of empowerment even in uncertain times.

Nature offers profound lessons in resilience and balance. Observing the cycles of the seasons, the persistence of a tree weathering a storm, or the adaptability of animals to their environments provides inspiration and perspective. Spending time in nature not only calms the nervous system but also reconnects individuals to the rhythms of life, reminding them of their own capacity to adapt and thrive.

The practice of resilience and balance is not without its challenges. Modern life often demands constant productivity and multitasking, leaving little room for rest or self-care. Social pressures and cultural narratives can make it difficult to prioritize balance without feeling guilt or inadequacy. However, holistic individuals approach these challenges with compassion and a commitment to living authentically, recognizing that their well-being is essential not only for themselves but also for those around them.

Examples of resilience and balance in action are both inspiring and relatable. A single parent juggling work and family responsibilities finds strength in mindfulness and gratitude, creating moments of joy amidst the chaos. An entrepreneur navigating setbacks uses journaling and self-reflection to adapt their vision and persevere. A teacher, balancing the demands of their profession, integrates restorative yoga and nature walks into their routine, replenishing their energy to better serve their students.

Ultimately, resilience and balance are not destinations but ongoing practices. They require attentiveness, adaptability, and a willingness to learn from both successes and setbacks. Each small step—whether taking a deep breath in a moment of stress, choosing to rest instead of overworking, or seeking support during difficult times—contributes to a life lived with intention and harmony.

Through resilience and balance, we cultivate the inner strength to face life's challenges and the wisdom to create a life of alignment. These practices remind us that even amidst uncertainty, we have the power to find peace, growth, and meaning. Together, resilience and balance illuminate the path to a holistic and fulfilling existence, guiding us toward our highest potential.

Chapter 16
The Inner Journey

The inner journey is a sacred path of self-discovery, healing, and transformation. It is an exploration of the soul's depths, a journey inward to uncover the truths, patterns, and desires that shape our lives. Unlike outward pursuits, which seek fulfillment in external achievements, the inner journey focuses on introspection and connection to one's authentic self. It is a deeply personal and transformative process that unfolds gradually, requiring courage, patience, and intention.

At the heart of the inner journey lies the question: *Who am I?* This timeless inquiry invites individuals to peel back the layers of social conditioning, roles, and expectations that often obscure their true essence. The inner journey is not about reaching a definitive answer but about embracing the process of self-discovery. It is a continuous unfolding, where each insight reveals deeper truths and new possibilities.

One of the first steps in the inner journey is cultivating awareness. This involves noticing thoughts, emotions, and behaviors without judgment, becoming an observer of one's inner world. Practices such as mindfulness meditation, journaling, and self-reflection help individuals tune into their inner dialogue and patterns. This awareness illuminates the subconscious beliefs and emotions that often drive actions, enabling intentional change.

As individuals embark on the inner journey, they often encounter limiting beliefs and emotional blockages. These are the stories and wounds that have accumulated over time, shaping how we perceive ourselves and the world. For example, someone might carry the belief that they are unworthy of love or success due to past experiences. The inner journey provides an opportunity to challenge these narratives, replacing them with affirming and empowering truths.

Shadow work is a pivotal aspect of the inner journey. Coined by Carl Jung, the shadow refers to the parts of ourselves that we suppress or reject, such as fears, insecurities, and unhealed wounds. These hidden aspects often manifest in unconscious behaviors, projections, or emotional triggers. By bringing the shadow into the light with compassion and acceptance, individuals integrate these aspects, reclaiming their wholeness.

Another essential element of the inner journey is exploring one's values and desires. What truly matters? What brings joy and fulfillment? By aligning actions and choices with these core values, individuals create a life that feels authentic and meaningful. This process requires honesty and the willingness to let go of societal expectations or obligations that no longer resonate.

The inner journey often involves facing discomfort and uncertainty. Healing past wounds, confronting fears, or embracing change can feel challenging and even overwhelming. However, these moments of difficulty are often the gateways to profound growth and transformation. The holistic perspective emphasizes that discomfort is not a sign of failure but a necessary part of the journey, an indicator that growth is occurring.

Creative expression is a powerful tool for navigating the inner journey. Writing, painting, music, and other forms of art allow individuals to explore and express their emotions and insights in ways that transcend words. These creative practices provide a safe and expansive space to process experiences, discover new perspectives, and connect with one's intuition.

Spiritual practices also play a significant role in the inner journey. Meditation, prayer, energy healing, or simply spending time in nature foster a sense of connection to something greater than oneself. These practices create a space of stillness and reflection, where deeper truths can emerge. They remind individuals that they are part of a larger whole, offering perspective and guidance along the path.

A particularly transformative aspect of the inner journey is the exploration of one's inner child. The inner child represents the part of us that carries the innocence, wonder, and vulnerabilities of childhood. Reconnecting with this aspect of the self often reveals unhealed wounds or unmet needs from early life. Through practices like visualization, dialogue, or therapy, individuals can nurture their inner child, providing the love and care they may have lacked.

The inner journey is not a solitary endeavor. While it is deeply personal, it is often supported by relationships, mentors, or communities. Trusted friends, therapists, or spiritual guides can provide encouragement, perspective, and accountability. Sharing the journey with others who are also on the path fosters connection and reminds us that we are not alone in our struggles or triumphs.

Rituals and practices can serve as anchors during the inner journey. Simple acts such as lighting a candle, creating a sacred space for reflection, or practicing gratitude rituals bring intention and focus to the process. These practices act as reminders of the commitment to self-discovery and the sacredness of the path.

As individuals progress on the inner journey, they begin to experience shifts in their external lives. Relationships deepen, priorities become clearer, and a sense of peace and fulfillment emerges. These changes are not the result of external circumstances but of the inner alignment that the journey cultivates.

The inner journey is also marked by moments of awakening—times when the world seems to shift, and clarity or inspiration arises. These moments may come during meditation, in nature, or unexpectedly during daily life. They provide glimpses of the interconnectedness and purpose that underpin existence, offering motivation to continue the journey.

One of the most profound lessons of the inner journey is the realization that growth is not linear. Progress is marked by cycles of expansion and contraction, clarity and confusion. There are times of profound insight and times of stillness or even stagnation. Embracing these cycles with patience and trust is key to navigating the journey with grace.

Stories of transformation illustrate the power of the inner journey. A person grappling with self-doubt begins a daily journaling practice, uncovering the roots of their insecurity and gradually building confidence. Another, recovering from grief, finds solace in meditation and nature, reconnecting with their sense of purpose. These journeys remind us that while the path may be challenging, it is also deeply rewarding.

Ultimately, the inner journey leads to a profound sense of self-acceptance and empowerment. It teaches us that the answers we seek are already within us, waiting to be uncovered through reflection and presence. It is a reminder that we are not defined by external circumstances or past experiences but by our capacity to learn, heal, and grow.

The inner journey is not a destination but a way of being. It invites us to approach life with curiosity, courage, and compassion, continually uncovering the layers of our authentic selves. Through this journey, we come to understand that the greatest discoveries lie not in the external world but in the vast and infinite universe within.

Chapter 17
Vibrations and Frequencies

The universe is composed of vibrations and frequencies, a symphony of energy that connects everything in existence. From the subatomic particles that form matter to the thoughts and emotions that shape our experiences, vibrations are the foundation of all that is. Understanding and working with these frequencies unlocks profound insights into health, emotions, and spiritual connection, offering a path to harmony and transformation.

Vibrations and frequencies are not abstract concepts—they are measurable phenomena that influence our physical, mental, and energetic states. Quantum physics reveals that everything, even the densest matter, is made up of energy vibrating at specific frequencies. Higher frequencies are associated with light, love, and positivity, while lower frequencies correlate with fear, anger, and negativity. By consciously raising our vibration, we align with states of well-being and abundance.

The human body, like the universe, is an energetic system. Each organ, cell, and system vibrates at a unique frequency, contributing to the body's overall energy field. When the body is in balance, these frequencies are harmonious, supporting health and vitality. However, stress, trauma, or negative emotions can disrupt this harmony, creating energetic blockages that manifest as physical illness or emotional distress.

One of the most direct ways to influence vibrations is through sound. Sound healing, an ancient practice found in cultures worldwide, harnesses specific frequencies to restore balance and harmony. Instruments like singing bowls, tuning forks, and gongs produce tones that resonate with the body's natural frequencies, clearing energetic blockages and promoting relaxation. For example, Tibetan singing bowls are tuned to specific notes that correspond to the body's chakras, aligning and harmonizing these energy centers.

Music, too, has a profound impact on vibrations. Listening to uplifting or soothing music raises one's frequency, evoking emotions like joy, peace, and inspiration. Conversely, harsh or dissonant sounds can lower vibrations, creating feelings of tension or unease. This awareness empowers individuals to curate their auditory environment, using music as a tool for emotional and energetic well-being.

The connection between emotions and vibrations is another key aspect of this phenomenon. Emotions like love, gratitude, and compassion resonate at high frequencies, while fear, shame, and anger vibrate at lower levels. By cultivating positive emotions, we elevate our vibration, enhancing our health, relationships, and spiritual connection. Practices like gratitude journaling, heart-centered meditation, and acts of kindness help shift emotional states and raise vibrational energy.

Thoughts, too, carry vibrational energy. Positive, affirming thoughts generate higher frequencies, attracting experiences that align with abundance and joy. Negative or self-limiting thoughts, on the other hand, create denser energy, perpetuating cycles of struggle or lack. Recognizing this dynamic, holistic individuals practice mindfulness and intentional thinking, using affirmations and visualization to align their mental energy with their highest aspirations.

The chakra system provides a framework for understanding how vibrations operate within the human body. Each chakra, or energy center, vibrates at a specific frequency and corresponds to physical, emotional, and spiritual aspects of life. For example, the heart chakra resonates with love and compassion, while the throat chakra vibrates with truth and communication. Imbalances in these energy centers can be addressed through practices like Reiki, sound healing, or visualization, restoring vibrational harmony.

Crystals and gemstones are another tool for working with vibrations. Each crystal carries a unique frequency that interacts with the body's energy field. Amethyst, for instance, vibrates at a frequency associated with calm and spiritual awareness, while citrine resonates with abundance and confidence. Wearing, carrying, or meditating with crystals allows individuals to harness these energies for healing and transformation.

Nature, too, is a powerful source of high-frequency energy. The rustling of leaves, the sound of ocean waves, and the stillness of a forest all resonate with frequencies that restore and rejuvenate. Spending time in nature not only calms the mind but also realigns the body's vibrations with the earth's natural rhythms. Practices like forest bathing, grounding (walking barefoot on the earth), and simply observing natural beauty amplify this connection.

Water, often referred to as the "universal conductor," plays a vital role in vibrations. Dr. Masaru Emoto's groundbreaking research demonstrated how the molecular structure of water changes in response to vibrational input. Positive words, music, and intentions create harmonious, crystalline patterns in water, while negative inputs create chaotic structures. As the human body is primarily composed of water, these findings emphasize the importance of surrounding ourselves with high-frequency energy.

The principle of resonance further illustrates how vibrations affect us. When two objects vibrate at different frequencies, the higher frequency can raise the vibration of the lower one, a phenomenon known as sympathetic resonance. This principle explains why spending time with uplifting people or engaging in activities that inspire joy elevates our own energy. Conversely, negative environments or interactions can lower our vibration, highlighting the need for conscious choices about where and with whom we spend our time.

Quantum physics also introduces the concept of entrainment, where systems in close proximity synchronize their frequencies over time. This principle is evident in human interactions, where emotions and energy are contagious. A calm, centered individual can bring stability to a chaotic situation, while anxiety can spread rapidly through a group. By maintaining high vibrations, holistic individuals positively influence their surroundings, creating ripples of harmony and peace.

Healing practices like acupuncture, Reiki, and energy work operate on the principle of restoring vibrational balance. These modalities focus on clearing blockages and realigning the body's energy field, allowing life force energy to flow freely. By addressing the energetic root of imbalances, these practices support both physical and emotional healing.

The role of intention cannot be overstated in working with vibrations and frequencies. Setting a clear, positive intention directs energy toward a desired outcome, amplifying its impact. Whether through prayer, visualization, or affirmation, intention acts as a vibrational blueprint, aligning the individual with their goals and aspirations.

Science continues to validate the impact of vibrations on health and well-being. Studies on brainwave frequencies, for example, reveal how different states of consciousness—such as relaxation, focus, or creativity—correlate with specific brainwave patterns. Practices like binaural beats and sound therapy harness these frequencies to enhance mental and emotional states.

The exploration of vibrations and frequencies is not confined to individual growth—it also extends to collective consciousness. When groups meditate, pray, or focus on positive intentions together, their combined energy creates a powerful vibrational field. This phenomenon has been observed in studies where mass meditation events reduce crime rates or promote peace in communities, demonstrating the potential of collective vibrational alignment.

Ultimately, understanding and working with vibrations and frequencies empower individuals to become conscious co-creators of their reality. By raising their vibration through thoughts, emotions, and actions, they align with states of health, abundance, and joy. This journey is not about achieving perfection but about cultivating awareness and intentionality in the energy we embody and share.

The universe, at its essence, is a vibrational dance of energy. By tuning into this rhythm, we reconnect with the flow of life, harmonizing with the frequencies that elevate and inspire. Through the exploration of vibrations and frequencies, we uncover the profound truth that we are not separate from the universe—we are its resonant song, an integral part of its infinite melody.

Chapter 18
Science and Holism

The relationship between science and holism is an evolving dialogue, bridging ancient wisdom and modern discoveries. For centuries, science and holistic traditions were perceived as opposites—science focused on breaking phenomena into measurable parts, while holism emphasized the interconnectedness of all things. Today, these perspectives are converging, as science begins to validate and illuminate principles long held by holistic traditions. This chapter explores how modern research is uncovering the mechanisms behind holistic practices, deepening our understanding of the mind, body, and universe.

Holism views the human experience as a dynamic interplay between physical, mental, emotional, and spiritual dimensions. Modern science, particularly in fields such as neuroscience, quantum physics, and psychoneuroimmunology, increasingly supports this integrative perspective. These disciplines reveal that the mind and body are not separate but deeply interconnected, and that the well-being of one profoundly influences the other.

One of the most compelling examples of this integration is the mind-body connection. Psychoneuroimmunology, the study of how thoughts and emotions affect the immune system, demonstrates that stress and negative emotions weaken the body's defenses, while positive states like gratitude and love enhance resilience. Practices such as meditation, mindfulness, and yoga, which have been central to holistic traditions for millennia, are now recognized for their ability to reduce stress, lower inflammation, and promote overall health.

The brain's plasticity, or neuroplasticity, is another area where science aligns with holistic principles. Neuroplasticity refers to the brain's ability to rewire itself in response to thoughts, behaviors, and experiences. This discovery validates the holistic practice of using affirmations, visualization, and mindfulness to shift mental patterns and create lasting change. Studies show that consistent meditation, for example, not only reduces stress but also increases gray matter in areas of the brain associated with emotional regulation and focus.

Quantum physics, too, provides insights that resonate with holistic perspectives. At the subatomic level, particles are not static but exist as waves of energy, interconnected and influenced by observation. This quantum reality parallels the holistic view that all things are interconnected and that intention shapes experience. Concepts such as quantum entanglement, where particles remain connected regardless of distance, mirror the idea of energetic unity found in many spiritual traditions.

The study of vibrations and frequencies further bridges science and holism. Sound therapy, for instance, uses specific frequencies to align the body's energy and promote healing. Research on brainwave frequencies shows how sound and meditation can induce states of relaxation, focus, and creativity by synchronizing the brain's activity. Tools such as binaural beats and singing bowls, long used in holistic practices, are now backed by studies demonstrating their physiological and psychological benefits.

Holistic nutrition is another area where science validates ancient practices. Research on the gut-brain connection reveals how the microbiome, the collection of bacteria in the digestive system, influences mood, cognition, and immunity. This aligns with the holistic view that food is medicine and that a balanced diet supports not just physical health but mental and emotional well-being. Foods rich in nutrients, such as leafy greens, berries, and fermented products, are shown to boost gut health and, in turn, improve mental clarity and emotional stability.

Energy healing practices, such as Reiki and acupuncture, are gaining scientific recognition as well. While the mechanisms behind these modalities remain partially understood, studies suggest that they influence the body's nervous system and biofield—a subtle energy field surrounding all living beings. Research shows that acupuncture can stimulate the release of endorphins and regulate the body's energy flow, while Reiki induces a state of deep relaxation, reducing stress and enhancing overall well-being.

Holistic approaches to movement, such as yoga and tai chi, also benefit from scientific exploration. Yoga, for example, has been shown to lower cortisol levels, improve flexibility, and increase strength, while also reducing symptoms of anxiety and depression. Tai chi, often described as "meditation in motion," improves balance, reduces stress, and enhances cardiovascular health. These practices highlight the holistic principle that movement is not just physical but also mental and energetic.

Heart coherence, a concept studied by the HeartMath Institute, demonstrates the science of emotional energy. When individuals experience positive emotions like love, gratitude, or compassion, the heart's rhythm becomes harmonious, creating a state of coherence that benefits both the body and mind. This state has been linked to improved immune function, emotional resilience, and enhanced problem-solving abilities. Such findings echo the holistic belief that the heart is a powerful center of energy and intuition.

Scientific research also supports the efficacy of mindfulness-based stress reduction (MBSR), a program developed to integrate mindfulness meditation into healthcare. Studies show that MBSR reduces symptoms of chronic pain, anxiety, and depression, while improving quality of life. This evidence-based approach brings holistic practices into mainstream medical settings, bridging the gap between ancient wisdom and modern medicine.

Environmental science offers another connection to holism, emphasizing the interconnectedness of humans and nature. Studies on biophilia, the innate human connection to nature, show that spending time outdoors reduces stress, lowers blood pressure, and enhances mood. Practices such as forest bathing, which originated in Japan, are now scientifically recognized for their ability to boost immunity and mental health, reinforcing the holistic principle that nature is a source of healing and balance.

The integration of science and holism extends to spirituality. Research on prayer and meditation shows their effects on the brain, including increased activity in areas associated with compassion and reduced activity in regions linked to fear. Near-death experiences and studies on consciousness challenge traditional scientific paradigms, suggesting that awareness may extend beyond the physical brain, aligning with holistic views of the soul and universal connection.

While science and holism are increasingly aligned, challenges remain. Holistic practices often operate in realms that are difficult to measure using traditional scientific methods. Energy fields, for example, elude standard instrumentation, leading to skepticism in mainstream science. However, advancements in technology and research are gradually expanding the boundaries of what can be studied, paving the way for greater integration.

The relationship between science and holism is not one of opposition but of complementarity. Science provides tools to explore and validate holistic practices, while holism offers a broader context that emphasizes connection, meaning, and purpose. Together, they create a more comprehensive understanding of health, well-being, and the nature of existence.

As science continues to explore the principles underlying holistic traditions, the gap between ancient wisdom and modern knowledge narrows. This convergence not only validates the efficacy of holistic practices but also enriches our understanding of the interconnected universe we inhabit.

Ultimately, the integration of science and holism reminds us that knowledge and wisdom are not static but evolving. By embracing both, we create a future where technology and tradition, logic and intuition, work together to foster a deeper connection to ourselves, each other, and the world around us. This union of perspectives empowers us to live more balanced, meaningful, and harmonious lives, guided by the best of both worlds.

Chapter 19
Connection with Nature

Nature is a profound source of balance, healing, and inspiration, offering a deep well of energy and wisdom for those who seek to connect with it. The holistic perspective recognizes that humans are not separate from nature but an integral part of its intricate web of life. This chapter explores the transformative power of connecting with the natural world and how it nurtures physical health, emotional well-being, and spiritual growth.

From the moment we take our first breath, nature sustains us. The air we breathe, the water we drink, and the food we consume are gifts of the earth. Yet, modern life often disconnects us from this symbiotic relationship, confining us to concrete cities, artificial environments, and fast-paced routines. Reconnecting with nature restores harmony, reminding us of our place within the larger ecosystem and grounding us in the rhythms of life.

One of the most accessible ways to connect with nature is through immersion in natural environments. Forest bathing, or *shinrin-yoku*, is a Japanese practice of spending intentional time in forests to absorb the healing benefits of the natural world. Studies have shown that walking among trees lowers cortisol levels, reduces blood pressure, and enhances mood. The gentle rustling of leaves, the earthy scent of soil, and the soothing light filtering through branches create a sensory experience that calms the mind and revitalizes the spirit.

Water, too, holds a unique power to heal and rejuvenate. Whether standing by the ocean, walking along a riverbank, or soaking in a natural spring, the presence of water has been shown to reduce stress and promote clarity. This phenomenon, often called the "blue mind effect," underscores the calming influence of water on the human psyche. The sound of waves or the sight of flowing streams reminds us of life's natural ebb and flow, encouraging us to let go of tension and embrace the present moment.

Gardening offers another intimate connection with nature. Planting seeds, tending to soil, and witnessing the growth of flowers, fruits, or vegetables fosters a sense of partnership with the earth. Gardening has been linked to reduced anxiety, improved mood, and a sense of accomplishment. It also serves as a powerful metaphor for personal growth, teaching patience, care, and the cycles of life and renewal.

For those seeking a deeper spiritual connection, nature provides an ideal setting for meditation and reflection. Sitting in stillness beneath a tree, gazing at the stars, or walking barefoot on the earth grounds the body and opens the mind to higher awareness. These practices cultivate a sense of oneness with the natural world, dissolving the illusion of separation and fostering a profound sense of interconnectedness.

Rituals in nature amplify this connection. Creating altars with natural elements, offering gratitude to the earth, or observing seasonal transitions are ways to honor the cycles of life and align with their energy. Many indigenous traditions emphasize these rituals, celebrating the solstices, equinoxes, and other natural phenomena as sacred moments of reflection and renewal.

Nature also teaches us through its cycles and resilience. The changing seasons reflect the rhythms of life—birth, growth, decline, and renewal. Observing these patterns reminds us to embrace life's transitions with grace, trusting that every ending holds the seed of a new beginning. Similarly, witnessing a tree thrive in harsh conditions or a flower bloom after a storm inspires resilience, reminding us of our own capacity to adapt and flourish.

The act of grounding, or earthing, is a simple yet profound way to connect with the earth's energy. Walking barefoot on grass, sand, or soil allows the body to absorb electrons from the earth, which help neutralize free radicals and reduce inflammation. Grounding also promotes emotional balance, providing a sense of stability and calm in the face of stress.

Nature's role in holistic health extends beyond emotional and spiritual well-being to include physical healing. Herbal medicine, for example, harnesses the therapeutic properties of plants to support the body's natural healing processes. From chamomile's calming effects to turmeric's anti-inflammatory benefits, plants have been used for millennia to treat ailments and enhance vitality.

Sustainable living practices deepen our connection with nature by fostering a sense of responsibility and care for the environment. Reducing waste, conserving water, and choosing eco-friendly products are not just acts of stewardship but expressions of gratitude for the earth's abundance. By living in alignment with nature's principles, we create a relationship that is reciprocal rather than extractive.

Spending time in nature also enhances creativity and problem-solving. Research shows that exposure to natural environments boosts cognitive function and inspires innovative thinking. The expansive vistas of mountains or the intricate patterns of a leaf awaken a sense of wonder, encouraging us to see the world—and our challenges—from fresh perspectives.

Children, in particular, benefit profoundly from time spent in nature. Outdoor play fosters physical health, creativity, and emotional resilience. It teaches children to observe, explore, and connect with the world around them, instilling a lifelong appreciation for the natural world. Programs like forest schools, which emphasize outdoor learning, demonstrate how nature-based education can enhance development and well-being.

For those who live in urban environments, connecting with nature may require creativity. Visiting parks, cultivating indoor plants, or simply observing the sky from a balcony can provide moments of connection. Even small acts, like tending to a windowsill herb garden or taking a lunch break in a green space, bring the benefits of nature into daily life.

The relationship between nature and humanity is reciprocal. Just as nature nourishes us, we are called to protect and honor it. This responsibility extends to addressing environmental challenges such as deforestation, pollution, and climate change. Holistic living emphasizes that our well-being is inseparable from the health of the planet, inspiring actions that contribute to sustainability and regeneration.

Stories of transformation highlight the profound impact of connecting with nature. A person recovering from burnout finds solace and clarity through daily walks in the woods. A community comes together to restore a local garden, fostering connection and purpose. A child struggling with anxiety discovers joy and confidence through outdoor exploration. These experiences remind us that nature is not merely a backdrop to life but an active participant in our journey.

Ultimately, connection with nature is a return to our roots—a reminder that we are not separate from the earth but deeply intertwined with its rhythms and energy. This connection grounds us in the present, nourishes our spirit, and inspires us to live in harmony with the world around us.

By embracing nature as a partner in our holistic journey, we rediscover the beauty and wisdom inherent in the natural world. We learn to listen to its rhythms, honor its gifts, and align our lives with its flow. In doing so, we cultivate a sense of belonging and balance, finding not only healing but also a profound sense of wonder and gratitude for the miracle of life.

Chapter 20
Healing Through Sound

Sound is one of the oldest and most powerful tools for healing, a universal language that transcends barriers and connects us to the rhythms of the universe. From the hum of a Tibetan singing bowl to the resonant tones of a human voice, sound carries frequencies that penetrate the body, mind, and spirit. This chapter explores the transformative potential of sound therapy and its ability to restore harmony, balance energy, and elevate consciousness.

At its core, sound healing is based on the principle that everything in the universe vibrates at a specific frequency, including the human body. When these frequencies fall out of balance due to stress, illness, or emotional upheaval, sound can act as a tuning fork, guiding the body and mind back into alignment. This practice is not new; ancient cultures around the world have used sound for centuries as a pathway to healing and transformation.

In Tibetan traditions, singing bowls are used to produce deep, resonant tones that calm the mind and harmonize the body's energy centers, or chakras. Similarly, in ancient Greece, Pythagoras explored the healing power of music and sound vibrations, using specific tones to bring balance to the body and emotions. Indigenous cultures have long employed drumming, chanting, and flute music in rituals, harnessing sound as a medium for spiritual connection and physical healing.

Modern sound therapy builds on these traditions, combining ancient wisdom with scientific understanding. Instruments such as crystal bowls, tuning forks, gongs, and chimes are carefully tuned to specific frequencies that resonate with the body's natural energy field. These frequencies can break up energetic blockages, release stagnant emotions, and promote relaxation and clarity.

The human voice is one of the most profound instruments of sound healing. Chanting, toning, and singing activate the body's vibrational field, releasing tension and promoting a sense of connection. Practices like *Om* chanting are particularly effective, as the sound of *Om* is believed to be the primordial vibration of the universe, aligning the individual with the cosmos.

One of the most researched aspects of sound healing is the use of binaural beats. This technique involves playing two slightly different frequencies in each ear, creating a third frequency perceived by the brain. This auditory illusion, known as the binaural beat, encourages the brain to synchronize its activity to the desired frequency, inducing states of relaxation, focus, or creativity. For example, low-frequency beats can guide the brain into a meditative state, while higher frequencies promote alertness and concentration.

Music therapy is another powerful form of sound healing, using melodies and rhythms to address physical, emotional, and cognitive challenges. Studies have shown that listening to or creating music reduces anxiety, improves mood, and even lowers blood pressure. For individuals with dementia, music therapy can evoke memories and enhance communication, reconnecting them with their sense of self and others.

Sound baths, a modern practice rooted in ancient techniques, immerse participants in a sea of healing vibrations. During a sound bath, practitioners use instruments like gongs, crystal bowls, and chimes to create layers of sound that wash over the body. This experience induces a deeply meditative state, where the mind quiets, and the body enters a state of profound relaxation and healing.

The science behind sound healing supports its efficacy. Sound waves travel through the body, penetrating tissues and stimulating cells. Studies have demonstrated that certain frequencies promote the production of nitric oxide, a molecule that relaxes blood vessels, enhances circulation, and boosts immune function. Additionally, sound vibrations can entrain brainwave activity, helping individuals shift from states of stress to calm or focus.

Chakra balancing is a common goal of sound healing, as each chakra corresponds to a specific frequency and element. For instance:

- The root chakra resonates with deep, grounding tones, often associated with drums or low-pitched instruments.
- The heart chakra aligns with soft, melodic sounds that evoke love and compassion, such as flutes or singing bowls tuned to the note F.
- The crown chakra, connected to higher consciousness, responds to ethereal, high-pitched sounds, fostering spiritual awakening.

Sound healing is also deeply connected to the emotional body. Many people experience emotional releases during sound therapy sessions, as vibrations dislodge suppressed feelings and bring them to the surface for healing. Crying, laughing, or feeling a sudden sense of peace are all common responses, reflecting the profound impact of sound on the subconscious mind.

One of the most remarkable aspects of sound healing is its accessibility. You don't need to be a trained musician or therapist to experience its benefits. Simple practices, such as humming, singing, or listening to nature sounds like rain or birdsong, can create a sense of calm and connection. Many people find that playing an instrument or singing intuitively becomes a form of meditation, allowing emotions to flow freely and energy to align.

For those seeking structured sound healing experiences, guided sound meditations and workshops provide opportunities for exploration. Online platforms and apps also offer access to binaural beats, soundscapes, and guided meditations, making sound healing more accessible than ever.

Incorporating sound healing into daily life is simple yet transformative. Starting the day with a brief chanting session, using soft music to unwind in the evening, or pausing to listen mindfully to the sounds of nature can shift your energy and mindset. These small practices create moments of harmony, reminding you of your connection to the universal vibration.

Stories of healing through sound are as diverse as the individuals who experience it. A person recovering from trauma finds solace and emotional release in the resonant tones of a gong. A stressed professional discovers clarity and focus by listening to binaural beats during meditation. A child with autism responds to the soothing melodies of a music therapist, enhancing communication and trust.

The healing power of sound extends beyond individuals to influence entire communities. Group chanting, drum circles, and sound healing ceremonies create collective energy fields that foster connection and unity. These shared experiences amplify the impact of sound, resonating not only within each participant but across the collective vibration of the group.

Ultimately, healing through sound is an invitation to remember our vibrational nature. It reminds us that we are part of a larger symphony, connected to the rhythms of the earth, the universe, and each other. Sound has the power to transcend the boundaries of language, culture, and even time, offering a universal pathway to balance and transformation.

By embracing the practice of sound healing, we open ourselves to the profound potential of vibration. We rediscover the harmony within and around us, aligning with the universal flow of life. In this resonance, we find not only healing but also a sense of wholeness—a reminder that, at our core, we are all expressions of the same infinite song.

Chapter 21
The Power of Gratitude

Gratitude is a transformative energy, a profound force that elevates the mind, heals the heart, and nurtures the soul. It shifts focus from what is lacking to what is abundant, creating a mindset of appreciation and positivity. For the holistic individual, gratitude is more than a fleeting emotion—it is a practice, a way of being that shapes how we experience the world.

At its essence, gratitude is the recognition of life's gifts, both big and small. It is the ability to see the beauty in a sunrise, the kindness in a stranger's gesture, or the lessons in a challenge. This awareness opens the heart, fostering connection and joy. Gratitude does not require perfect circumstances; instead, it invites us to find value in the present moment, regardless of its imperfections.

The power of gratitude lies in its ability to rewire the brain. Neuroscience reveals that regular gratitude practice activates regions of the brain associated with happiness and emotional regulation, such as the prefrontal cortex and the hypothalamus. Over time, this strengthens neural pathways, making gratitude a natural and automatic response. It also increases the release of dopamine and serotonin, the brain's "feel-good" chemicals, enhancing overall well-being.

One of the most effective ways to cultivate gratitude is through journaling. Writing down three to five things you are grateful for each day helps shift focus toward the positive aspects of life. These can range from profound experiences, like reconnecting with a loved one, to simple pleasures, like the warmth of the sun or the taste of a favorite meal. The act of writing deepens the practice, solidifying gratitude as a habit.

Gratitude meditation is another powerful tool. This practice involves sitting in stillness and bringing to mind people, experiences, or things for which you are thankful. Visualizing these sources of gratitude and feeling the accompanying emotions enhances the connection to this energy. Gratitude meditation not only calms the mind but also opens the heart, fostering a sense of peace and fulfillment.

Acts of gratitude, such as expressing thanks to others, amplify its impact. A heartfelt note, a kind word, or a genuine acknowledgment strengthens relationships and spreads positivity. These expressions create a ripple effect, inspiring gratitude in others and fostering a culture of appreciation. Research shows that people who regularly express gratitude have stronger social connections, greater empathy, and increased resilience.

Gratitude also serves as a powerful antidote to negativity and stress. In challenging times, it may seem counterintuitive to focus on what is good, yet this is when gratitude is most transformative. By intentionally seeking out silver linings or lessons within difficulties, we shift our perspective from victimhood to empowerment. This does not diminish the reality of pain but provides a framework for moving through it with strength and hope.

In the holistic view, gratitude extends beyond the personal to encompass the collective and the universal. It invites us to honor the interconnectedness of all things—the earth that sustains us, the ancestors who paved the way, and the communities that support us. Expressing gratitude to nature, for example, deepens our bond with the environment, inspiring sustainable practices and care for the planet.

Spiritual traditions worldwide emphasize gratitude as a path to enlightenment. In Buddhism, gratitude cultivates awareness of life's interdependence. In Christianity, it is expressed as praise and thanksgiving to the divine. Indigenous practices often center on gratitude rituals, offering thanks to the earth, sky, and spirit for their gifts. These teachings highlight gratitude's spiritual dimension, reminding us of our place within the greater whole.

Gratitude rituals can enhance daily life. Beginning the day by reflecting on what you are thankful for sets a positive tone, while ending the day with a gratitude practice brings closure and peace. Some people create gratitude jars, writing down moments of appreciation and revisiting them during difficult times. These rituals anchor the practice of gratitude, making it a consistent part of life.

The power of gratitude is not limited to individuals; it has the potential to transform communities and societies. When gratitude becomes a shared value, it fosters collaboration, trust, and mutual respect. Organizations that prioritize gratitude—through recognition programs, acts of appreciation, or supportive cultures—experience greater employee satisfaction, loyalty, and productivity.

Gratitude also holds a profound energy for healing. It helps release resentment, anger, and bitterness, creating space for forgiveness and peace. In relationships, expressing gratitude for a partner's strengths and contributions strengthens bonds and rekindles connection. In self-healing, gratitude shifts focus from flaws to strengths, fostering self-acceptance and confidence.

The practice of gratitude even impacts physical health. Studies show that individuals who regularly cultivate gratitude have lower blood pressure, stronger immune systems, and better sleep quality. The connection between gratitude and physical well-being underscores the holistic principle that mind, body, and spirit are deeply intertwined.

Children, too, benefit from learning gratitude. Teaching them to say thank you, recognize acts of kindness, and appreciate the world around them instills a lifelong habit. Activities like creating gratitude trees, where children write what they are thankful for on leaves, make the practice tangible and engaging. These lessons foster empathy, humility, and happiness from an early age.

Stories of transformation through gratitude illustrate its power. A person battling illness finds strength and hope by focusing on the love and support of family. An entrepreneur facing setbacks rediscovers purpose by appreciating the journey rather than fixating on outcomes. A teacher struggling with burnout rekindles their passion by reflecting on the impact they've made on their students.

Gratitude is a bridge between the present and the infinite. It grounds us in the here and now while opening our hearts to the abundance of life. It teaches us that joy is not found in what we lack but in recognizing and celebrating what we already have.

Ultimately, gratitude is an act of alignment—with ourselves, with others, and with the universe. It invites us to live in harmony, honoring the gifts of existence and sharing them with the world. Through gratitude, we cultivate a life of meaning, connection, and boundless possibility.

The power of gratitude is its simplicity. It requires no special tools or conditions, only an open heart and a willingness to see. In every moment, gratitude is waiting, ready to transform how we perceive, experience, and live. It is a quiet but profound force, a reminder that life itself is the greatest gift of all.

Chapter 22
Rhythms and Cycles

Life is governed by rhythms and cycles, intricate patterns that echo through the natural world, our bodies, and the universe. From the phases of the moon to the beating of our hearts, these cycles provide a framework for harmony, growth, and renewal. By aligning with these rhythms, we reconnect with the flow of life, fostering balance, resilience, and a deeper understanding of our place within the cosmos.

At the foundation of these rhythms are the cycles of nature. The changing seasons, the tides, and the movement of celestial bodies all serve as reminders of life's constant flux. Spring brings renewal and growth, summer offers abundance and vitality, autumn invites reflection and release, and winter nurtures rest and introspection. These cycles encourage us to embrace change as a natural and necessary part of life.

The lunar cycle is one of the most profound rhythms that influence human experience. Each phase of the moon carries distinct energies that affect emotions, creativity, and focus. The new moon, for example, symbolizes beginnings and introspection, making it an ideal time for setting intentions and planting seeds for the future. The full moon, with its heightened energy, encourages completion, celebration, and the release of what no longer serves us. By observing these phases, individuals can align their actions and emotions with the natural ebb and flow of lunar energy.

In addition to external rhythms, the human body is attuned to its own cycles. The circadian rhythm, our internal clock, regulates sleep, energy levels, and bodily functions over a 24-

hour period. Disruptions to this rhythm, such as irregular sleep patterns or exposure to artificial light, can lead to fatigue, stress, and imbalances in health. Practices like maintaining consistent sleep schedules, reducing screen time before bed, and spending time in natural sunlight help restore this vital cycle.

For women, the menstrual cycle is another powerful rhythm that influences physical, emotional, and energetic states. Each phase of the cycle—menstruation, the follicular phase, ovulation, and the luteal phase—offers unique opportunities for reflection, creativity, and growth. Honoring these phases, rather than resisting them, fosters a deeper connection to the body's wisdom and rhythms.

Breath, too, is a rhythm that sustains and centers us. Each inhale and exhale mirrors the cycles of expansion and contraction found throughout life. Breathwork practices, such as conscious breathing or pranayama, help regulate the nervous system, balance emotions, and create a sense of presence. By tuning into the rhythm of the breath, individuals find calm amidst chaos and clarity amidst confusion.

In holistic living, rhythms extend to daily, weekly, and seasonal practices that align with natural cycles. Morning rituals, for instance, harness the energy of a new day, fostering focus and intention. Evening routines create space for reflection and rest, honoring the need for balance. Weekly rhythms, such as dedicating time to creativity, social connection, or solitude, ensure that life remains fulfilling and dynamic.

Rituals tied to seasonal transitions deepen our connection to nature and its cycles. Spring rituals might involve planting seeds or decluttering spaces, reflecting the season's themes of renewal. Summer invites celebration and community, with activities that embrace vitality and abundance. Autumn encourages letting go, whether through journaling, releasing old habits, or clearing physical spaces. Winter nurtures introspection, with rituals like candlelight meditations or cozy evenings of rest and reflection.

The concept of rhythm also extends to work and productivity. The modern world often emphasizes constant output, ignoring the natural cycles of effort and rest. Aligning work habits with ultradian rhythms—periods of heightened focus followed by the need for a short break—enhances efficiency and prevents burnout. For example, the Pomodoro Technique, which alternates 25 minutes of focused work with 5-minute breaks, mirrors these natural cycles.

Music is a powerful way to connect with rhythms. The beat of a drum, the melody of a song, or the flow of a symphony resonates deeply with our inner rhythms, evoking emotions and memories. Dancing to music, whether alone or in community, allows individuals to express and release energy, syncing their movements with the universal flow.

Nature itself teaches us the importance of honoring cycles. Trees shed their leaves in autumn, animals hibernate in winter, and rivers flow at varying speeds depending on the season. These patterns remind us that rest is as vital as action, and that growth often occurs in cycles of effort followed by renewal.

Aligning with rhythms and cycles also fosters patience and trust. Just as a farmer trusts that planted seeds will grow in their own time, individuals learn to embrace the pace of their personal journeys. This perspective reduces the need for control and fosters a sense of harmony with life's unfolding.

In relationships, recognizing and honoring cycles of closeness and independence strengthens bonds. Just as the moon waxes and wanes, relationships thrive when they allow space for connection and individuality. This balance creates resilience, ensuring that partnerships remain dynamic and supportive over time.

The role of cycles in emotional healing is particularly profound. Emotions often arise in waves, building in intensity before subsiding. Allowing these cycles to unfold, rather than resisting or suppressing them, creates space for processing and release. Techniques like mindfulness, journaling, or somatic practices help individuals navigate these emotional rhythms with compassion and awareness.

Spiritual practices also align with rhythms and cycles. Meditating during the quiet hours of dawn, practicing gratitude at sunset, or observing rituals during the solstices and equinoxes connects individuals to the greater flow of life. These practices create a sense of sacredness in daily life, reminding us of our place within the cosmic rhythm.

Incorporating rhythms and cycles into holistic living requires attentiveness and intention. Keeping a journal to track energy levels, emotions, or lunar phases reveals personal patterns and preferences. Observing nature, whether through gardening, hiking, or simply sitting outdoors, deepens awareness of the cycles unfolding around us.

Stories of transformation through alignment with rhythms highlight their power. A busy professional finds renewed energy by honoring their circadian rhythm, establishing consistent sleep and work patterns. A woman reconnects with her inner strength by aligning her self-care practices with her menstrual cycle. A family strengthens their bond by celebrating seasonal rituals, fostering a sense of continuity and connection.

Ultimately, rhythms and cycles are a reminder that life is not linear but cyclical. Growth, rest, change, and renewal are natural and necessary parts of existence. By aligning with these patterns, we cultivate balance, resilience, and a sense of harmony with ourselves and the world.

In honoring rhythms and cycles, we embrace the wisdom of the universe. We learn to flow with life's natural currents, trusting the process and finding beauty in every phase. This alignment nurtures not only our well-being but also our connection to the greater whole, reminding us that we are part of an eternal, ever-unfolding rhythm.

Chapter 23
Emotions and Energy

Emotions are powerful forces that shape our experiences, influence our actions, and color our perceptions of the world. They are not just fleeting feelings but energetic vibrations that ripple through our bodies, minds, and souls. In holistic living, understanding the connection between emotions and energy is key to achieving balance, healing, and transformation. By learning to recognize, honor, and transmute emotional energy, we unlock the ability to live with greater clarity and alignment.

Emotions are energy in motion. They arise in response to our interactions, thoughts, and environment, and they carry a unique vibrational frequency. Positive emotions such as joy, gratitude, and love resonate at high frequencies, elevating our energy and contributing to physical and emotional well-being. Conversely, emotions like fear, anger, and sadness vibrate at lower frequencies, creating heaviness and, if left unprocessed, contributing to energetic blockages.

The body acts as a vessel for emotional energy, storing unresolved emotions in tissues, muscles, and cells. This is why unexpressed or repressed emotions often manifest as physical discomfort or illness. For example, chronic stress can lead to tension in the shoulders or digestive issues, while unresolved grief may linger as fatigue or chest tightness. Recognizing these physical manifestations is the first step in understanding the energy behind emotions.

Awareness is the cornerstone of emotional energy work. By observing emotions without judgment, we create space to understand their origin and message. Emotions are not inherently good or bad—they are simply signals, guiding us to pay attention to our inner world. Fear, for instance, may alert us to potential danger or an unresolved past trauma, while anger may signal a boundary that has been crossed.

Processing emotional energy requires intentional practices. Breathwork is a powerful tool for releasing stagnant emotions and restoring energetic flow. Deep, rhythmic breathing calms the nervous system, oxygenates the body, and helps move energy through areas of tension. Techniques such as diaphragmatic breathing or alternate nostril breathing bring immediate relief, shifting the body from a state of stress to one of balance.

Movement is another effective way to release emotional energy. Physical activities like yoga, dance, or even a brisk walk help dissipate the heaviness of emotions and create space for new energy to flow. Practices like shaking or intuitive movement allow the body to express emotions in a natural, uninhibited way, bypassing the analytical mind and reaching the core of emotional release.

Journaling provides a reflective space to explore emotions and their energetic impact. By putting thoughts and feelings into words, we externalize them, gaining perspective and insight. Journaling can also reveal patterns, such as recurring triggers or habitual reactions, enabling us to address underlying causes rather than surface symptoms.

Energy healing modalities such as Reiki, acupuncture, and EFT (Emotional Freedom Techniques) work directly with the body's energy field to balance and clear emotional blockages. These practices align the body's energy centers, or chakras, promoting harmony and releasing suppressed emotions. For example, the heart chakra, associated with love and forgiveness, may feel blocked after a painful breakup but can be reopened through targeted energy work and self-compassion.

Mindfulness meditation is a cornerstone practice for navigating emotions and energy. By bringing attention to the present moment, mindfulness helps us witness emotions as they arise, without becoming overwhelmed or entangled in them. Techniques such as body scans or loving-kindness meditations cultivate awareness and compassion, creating a safe container for emotional exploration.

Transmuting emotions involves shifting their energy from a lower vibration to a higher one. This process does not deny or suppress emotions but transforms their frequency. For example, anger can be channeled into assertive action, fear into curiosity, and sadness into creative expression. Visualization techniques, such as imagining a heavy emotion dissolving into light, help facilitate this energetic shift.

Gratitude is a powerful tool for raising emotional vibrations. Even in moments of difficulty, finding something to be grateful for shifts focus from lack to abundance. Gratitude elevates energy, creating a ripple effect that influences thoughts, feelings, and actions. Keeping a gratitude journal or pausing to acknowledge blessings throughout the day fosters a positive emotional baseline.

Boundaries play a crucial role in maintaining emotional and energetic balance. Recognizing when external influences drain energy allows us to protect our emotional well-being. Setting boundaries might involve limiting time with toxic individuals, saying no to overcommitments, or creating space for solitude and self-care. Healthy boundaries ensure that our energy remains centered and aligned.

Understanding the energetic nature of emotions also enhances relationships. By cultivating empathy and active listening, we create space for others to express their emotions without judgment. This exchange of emotional energy deepens connection and trust, fostering mutual support and understanding. It also teaches us to distinguish between our own emotions and those we absorb from others, enabling us to navigate relationships with clarity and compassion.

The role of forgiveness in emotional energy work cannot be overstated. Holding onto resentment or grudges creates energetic stagnation, while forgiveness frees us from the weight of the past. Forgiveness is not about condoning harm but about releasing its hold on our hearts. Practices like Ho'oponopono, a Hawaiian prayer of reconciliation, facilitate forgiveness by focusing on love, gratitude, and healing.

Children, too, benefit from understanding emotions as energy. Teaching them to name and express their feelings fosters emotional intelligence and resilience. Activities like drawing, storytelling, or breathing exercises help children process their emotions in healthy ways, preventing them from becoming internalized or overwhelming.

Stories of transformation through emotional energy work highlight its profound impact. A person burdened by grief finds release through journaling and meditation, reclaiming joy and purpose. An individual struggling with anger learns to channel it into advocacy, turning frustration into meaningful action. A couple navigating conflict discovers the power of empathy and active listening, strengthening their bond.

Ultimately, emotions are not obstacles but guides, leading us to greater self-awareness and alignment. They teach us about our needs, values, and desires, offering a roadmap for personal growth. By embracing emotions as energy, we reclaim our power to shape our inner and outer worlds.

The connection between emotions and energy reminds us of the dynamic, ever-changing nature of life. Just as waves rise and fall, emotions flow through us, inviting us to feel, release, and renew. By honoring this flow, we create harmony within ourselves and with the world around us, living with openness, courage, and balance.

Chapter 24
Radical Self-Acceptance

Radical self-acceptance is a profound act of transformation, one that embraces every part of who we are without condition or judgment. In a world that often promotes comparison, perfectionism, and external validation, self-acceptance offers a path to inner peace and authenticity. It is not a passive resignation but an active, courageous process of embracing both our light and shadow, reclaiming our wholeness, and stepping into our power.

At its core, radical self-acceptance is about recognizing that we are enough exactly as we are. It begins with releasing the idea that our worth is tied to achievements, appearances, or the approval of others. Instead, it invites us to honor our unique journey, flaws, and strengths as integral aspects of our being. This shift in perspective creates a foundation of self-compassion and resilience, allowing us to navigate life with greater confidence and ease.

The journey toward self-acceptance often requires unlearning societal and personal conditioning. From a young age, we absorb messages about how we "should" look, act, or succeed, shaping a narrative of inadequacy when we fall short of these expectations. Radical self-acceptance challenges these narratives, asking us to question who we are outside of these imposed standards.

Self-awareness is the first step in this process. By observing our thoughts, behaviors, and emotions without judgment, we begin to uncover the beliefs and patterns that undermine self-acceptance. Practices like mindfulness meditation, journaling, or introspective therapy provide tools for this exploration, creating space for honest self-reflection.

One of the most significant obstacles to self-acceptance is the inner critic—a voice that perpetuates doubt, shame, and self-judgment. This voice often stems from past experiences or unmet needs, internalized over time. Addressing the inner critic requires recognizing its presence, understanding its origins, and responding with compassion rather than hostility. Affirmations, self-kindness, and positive self-talk help to quiet this voice and replace it with one of support and encouragement.

Shadow work is another transformative tool for radical self-acceptance. The shadow represents the aspects of ourselves that we suppress or deny, often out of fear or shame. By bringing these parts into the light, we integrate them into our identity, reclaiming the energy spent hiding or avoiding them. For example, acknowledging feelings of jealousy or anger allows us to understand their roots and transform them into insights or strengths.

Forgiveness, both of self and others, is a cornerstone of self-acceptance. Holding onto regret, guilt, or resentment creates emotional barriers that prevent us from embracing who we are. Forgiving ourselves for past mistakes or perceived shortcomings is not about erasing them but about accepting that imperfection is part of the human experience. Similarly, forgiving others releases the hold of external judgments, freeing us to live authentically.

Body acceptance is a critical aspect of radical self-acceptance in a culture that often equates worth with physical appearance. Embracing one's body as it is—without comparison or criticism—cultivates a sense of gratitude and respect for its unique form and function. Practices like body positivity, intuitive movement, and mindfulness help shift the focus from appearance to the body's inherent wisdom and strength.

The role of vulnerability in self-acceptance cannot be overstated. Allowing ourselves to be seen as we truly are, without masks or pretense, fosters deeper connections and liberates us from the fear of rejection. Vulnerability is an act of courage, a declaration that our authenticity is more valuable than the illusion of perfection.

Gratitude and self-celebration further enhance self-acceptance. Taking time to acknowledge personal achievements, qualities, and growth—no matter how small—reinforces a sense of worthiness. Creating a gratitude practice focused on self-appreciation, such as listing three things you love about yourself each day, shifts the narrative from self-criticism to self-affirmation.

Boundaries are essential in protecting and nurturing self-acceptance. Recognizing and communicating limits ensures that relationships and commitments align with our values and well-being. Boundaries are acts of self-respect, signaling to ourselves and others that our needs and feelings matter.

Community also plays a role in fostering self-acceptance. Surrounding ourselves with supportive, compassionate individuals creates a safe space for authenticity. Sharing experiences, challenges, and triumphs with like-minded people reminds us that we are not alone in our struggles or growth.

Radical self-acceptance is particularly transformative during times of failure or change. Rather than viewing setbacks as reflections of inadequacy, this perspective reframes them as opportunities for learning and evolution. It encourages us to approach challenges with curiosity and resilience, trusting that our worth remains constant regardless of external circumstances.

The concept of self-acceptance extends to embracing life's dualities—strength and vulnerability, joy and sorrow, light and shadow. It is about acknowledging that we are multifaceted beings, capable of growth and contradiction. This holistic view fosters inner harmony, reducing the need for internal conflict or self-denial.

Teaching self-acceptance to children lays the foundation for lifelong resilience and self-esteem. Encouraging them to explore their interests, express their emotions, and embrace their individuality instills a sense of worthiness from an early age.

Modeling self-acceptance as adults further reinforces these values, creating an environment of acceptance and love.

The journey toward radical self-acceptance is not linear. It is a practice, one that requires patience, dedication, and self-compassion. There will be moments of doubt, resistance, or setback, but each step forward strengthens the foundation of self-love.

Stories of transformation highlight the profound impact of radical self-acceptance. An individual struggling with perfectionism learns to embrace their flaws, discovering greater creativity and joy in the process. A person burdened by past mistakes finds freedom through self-forgiveness, reclaiming their sense of worth. A parent navigating self-doubt models self-compassion for their child, creating a ripple effect of acceptance across generations.

Ultimately, radical self-acceptance is a return to wholeness. It is the recognition that we are already complete, that our value is inherent and unchanging. This acceptance allows us to move through life with authenticity, courage, and peace, unburdened by the need to prove or perfect.

In embracing radical self-acceptance, we unlock the potential for deeper connections, greater resilience, and a life lived in alignment with our true selves. It is an act of liberation, a declaration that we are enough, just as we are—a powerful truth that transforms not only how we see ourselves but also how we engage with the world.

Chapter 25
Simplicity and Essence

In a world increasingly defined by complexity and consumption, the pursuit of simplicity offers a pathway to clarity, peace, and alignment with one's true essence. Simplicity is not merely about reducing possessions or activities; it is about uncovering what truly matters and letting go of anything that distracts from it. It is a practice of intentional living that nurtures balance, joy, and a deep connection to oneself and the present moment.

At its core, simplicity is an act of discernment. It invites us to pause and reflect on what adds meaning and value to our lives, as opposed to what merely fills space or drains energy. This process begins with a question: What is essential? Answering this question requires honesty and courage, as it often challenges societal norms, habits, and attachments.

The philosophy of simplicity is rooted in the understanding that less is often more. By paring down, we create space for what truly enriches us—be it relationships, creativity, self-care, or inner peace. Simplicity frees us from the overwhelm of excess, allowing us to engage more fully with life.

Decluttering physical spaces is one of the most tangible ways to embrace simplicity. By letting go of items that no longer serve a purpose or bring joy, we create environments that feel open, organized, and calming. Minimalism, a practice of owning only what is essential, offers a framework for this process. However, simplicity is not about deprivation—it is about surrounding ourselves with things that align with our values and bring genuine satisfaction.

Beyond the physical, simplicity also applies to our mental and emotional spaces. The mind, like a cluttered room, can become overwhelmed by too many thoughts, obligations, or distractions. Practices like mindfulness meditation, journaling, and setting boundaries help clear this mental clutter, creating clarity and focus. By simplifying our mental and emotional lives, we cultivate a sense of calm and presence.

Time, too, is a resource that benefits from simplification. The modern tendency to overcommit and multitask often leads to stress and burnout. Simplicity encourages us to prioritize activities that align with our values and let go of unnecessary obligations. This might mean saying no to demands that do not serve us, creating buffer zones in our schedules, or dedicating time to rest and reflection.

The practice of simplicity is deeply tied to living in alignment with one's essence. Our essence is the core of who we are—our values, passions, and purpose. When we strip away external noise and distractions, we reconnect with this essence, gaining clarity about what truly matters. This alignment fosters authenticity and a sense of fulfillment, as our choices reflect our deepest truths.

Simplicity also extends to relationships. It encourages us to focus on quality over quantity, nurturing connections that are meaningful and supportive. Letting go of toxic or superficial relationships creates space for deeper, more authentic bonds. By practicing honest communication and presence in our interactions, we enrich the relationships that matter most.

In the context of work and productivity, simplicity emphasizes doing less but with greater focus and intention. Practices like single-tasking—focusing on one task at a time—enhance efficiency and reduce stress. Similarly, prioritizing tasks based on their alignment with long-term goals ensures that our efforts are meaningful rather than scattered.

Simplicity often involves reevaluating our relationship with material possessions. The modern consumer culture encourages accumulation, equating success with the number of things we own. However, studies show that material wealth does not necessarily lead to happiness. Instead, experiences—such as travel, learning, or time spent with loved ones—offer lasting fulfillment. By shifting our focus from owning to experiencing, we align with the principles of simplicity and essence.

Nature serves as a powerful teacher of simplicity. A tree does not accumulate more leaves than it needs; a river flows without excess. Spending time in nature reminds us of the beauty of simplicity, encouraging us to adopt its effortless harmony. Practices like gardening, hiking, or simply sitting outdoors connect us to this natural rhythm, grounding us in the present moment.

Simplicity also cultivates gratitude. When we strip away the excess, we become more attuned to the beauty and abundance of what remains. A simple meal, a quiet moment, or a heartfelt conversation takes on greater significance, fostering a sense of appreciation and contentment.

Minimalism is often associated with simplicity, but the two are not synonymous. Minimalism focuses on reducing possessions, while simplicity is a broader philosophy that encompasses all aspects of life—physical, emotional, mental, and spiritual. While minimalism can be a pathway to simplicity, it is not the only one. Each individual's approach to simplicity is unique, shaped by their values and circumstances.

One of the greatest benefits of simplicity is the freedom it brings. Letting go of what no longer serves us—whether material, emotional, or mental—liberates energy and attention for what truly matters. This freedom allows us to live more intentionally, focusing on what aligns with our essence and brings joy.

The journey toward simplicity is not about achieving perfection but about continuous refinement. It is a process of regularly reassessing what is essential and making adjustments as needed. Life's circumstances and priorities evolve, and simplicity invites us to adapt while remaining grounded in our values.

Teaching simplicity to children fosters resilience and creativity. Encouraging them to appreciate experiences over possessions, embrace stillness, and focus on what brings them joy helps build a foundation for intentional living. Modeling simplicity as adults further reinforces these lessons, creating an environment where simplicity is valued and celebrated.

Stories of transformation illustrate the power of simplicity. A professional overwhelmed by obligations finds balance by simplifying their schedule, prioritizing time for family and self-care. An individual seeking clarity declutters their home, creating a serene space that reflects their values. A couple embraces minimalism, reducing financial stress and deepening their connection through shared experiences.

Ultimately, simplicity is a return to essence. It is the recognition that we do not need to chase or accumulate to find fulfillment; everything we need is already within us. By embracing simplicity, we align with the flow of life, finding peace, clarity, and joy in the process.

In the practice of simplicity, we uncover the truth that life's beauty lies not in its complexity but in its essence. By letting go of the unnecessary, we create space for the extraordinary, reconnecting with ourselves, others, and the world in a way that is intentional, authentic, and deeply fulfilling.

Chapter 26
Global Connection

In an increasingly interconnected world, the holistic perspective emphasizes that we are not isolated individuals but part of a vast, dynamic web of relationships that span cultures, ecosystems, and generations. Global connection is more than technological or economic—it is a recognition of our shared humanity and the responsibility we have to one another and the planet. This chapter explores how the principles of holism inspire a sense of global unity, fostering collaboration, compassion, and collective action.

The foundation of global connection lies in the understanding that all life is interdependent. What affects one part of the system ultimately impacts the whole. This truth is evident in nature, where the health of an ecosystem depends on the balance and cooperation of its components. Similarly, humanity's well-being is tied to the health of the earth, the strength of our communities, and the equity of our societies.

Technology has revolutionized the way we connect globally, shrinking distances and enabling instant communication. Platforms for social media, virtual collaboration, and global learning have created opportunities to share ideas, build relationships, and address challenges collectively. However, while technology facilitates connection, it also highlights the importance of using these tools mindfully. Holistic living encourages us to approach digital spaces with intention, ensuring that they foster understanding and unity rather than division.

Global connection begins with empathy—the ability to see the world through another's eyes and feel compassion for their experiences. Empathy bridges cultural and societal differences, reminding us of our shared humanity. Practices like active listening, cultural exchange, and storytelling deepen this understanding, fostering mutual respect and reducing prejudice.

Community initiatives that prioritize global connection often emphasize collaboration and shared purpose. Grassroots movements, international organizations, and local groups working for environmental sustainability, social justice, or humanitarian aid demonstrate the power of collective action. These efforts not only address pressing issues but also build networks of trust and solidarity across borders.

One of the most pressing aspects of global connection is environmental stewardship. The health of the planet is a shared responsibility, requiring coordinated efforts to combat climate change, protect biodiversity, and promote sustainable practices. Initiatives like reforestation projects, renewable energy programs, and conservation efforts illustrate how global collaboration can lead to meaningful change. Holistic principles remind us that caring for the earth is not separate from caring for ourselves—it is an act of self-preservation and reverence for life.

Education plays a vital role in fostering global connection. Schools and programs that incorporate global perspectives teach students to appreciate cultural diversity, understand global challenges, and see themselves as citizens of the world. Holistic education emphasizes experiential learning, such as studying different cultures, participating in exchange programs, or engaging in community service, to build empathy and broaden perspectives.

Global connection also extends to economic practices. Holistic economics prioritizes fairness, sustainability, and the well-being of people and the planet. Supporting ethical businesses, fair trade initiatives, and local artisans contributes to equitable global systems. Additionally, mindfulness in consumption—buying only what is needed and choosing products with minimal environmental impact—aligns with the principles of global responsibility.

Art and culture are powerful tools for fostering global connection. Music, literature, visual arts, and dance transcend language barriers, conveying universal emotions and stories. Cultural exchanges and collaborations celebrate diversity while highlighting commonalities, creating a sense of shared humanity. By engaging with art from around the world, individuals gain insight into the experiences and perspectives of others, enriching their own understanding.

Spiritual traditions also emphasize the interconnectedness of all beings. Concepts like *ubuntu* from African philosophy, which translates to "I am because we are," or the Buddhist idea of interbeing reflect the holistic view that individual well-being is inseparable from collective well-being. These teachings inspire actions rooted in compassion, service, and unity, encouraging individuals to contribute positively to the global community.

Mindfulness practices, when applied to global connection, encourage awareness of how our choices impact others and the planet. For example, considering the environmental and social consequences of purchasing habits, travel, or energy use fosters a sense of accountability. This mindfulness transforms everyday actions into expressions of care and respect for the greater whole.

Language, though diverse, is another bridge for connection. Learning a new language or even a few words from another culture fosters respect and builds relationships. Language embodies history, values, and ways of thinking, and engaging with it opens doors to deeper understanding and appreciation.

The COVID-19 pandemic illustrated both the challenges and opportunities of global connection. While physical distancing and travel restrictions highlighted the vulnerabilities of a connected world, they also inspired unprecedented collaboration in science, healthcare, and mutual aid. The pandemic underscored the importance of solidarity, adaptability, and compassion in addressing global crises.

Global connection also requires addressing historical and systemic inequities. Holistic living calls for acknowledging the impact of colonization, racism, and economic disparity and working toward reconciliation and justice. This involves listening to marginalized voices, advocating for equity, and creating systems that uplift rather than exploit.

Storytelling is a particularly powerful medium for fostering global connection. Documentaries, memoirs, and oral histories bring to life the experiences of people from different cultures and backgrounds. By sharing these stories, we cultivate empathy and understanding, breaking down stereotypes and fostering a sense of unity.

For individuals seeking to deepen their global connection, small actions can create meaningful impact. Supporting local and global charities, volunteering for causes, and participating in cultural events are ways to contribute. Even small gestures, such as engaging in conversations with people from different backgrounds or learning about global issues, expand awareness and foster connection.

Children, too, benefit from learning about global connection. Encouraging curiosity about other cultures, teaching kindness, and involving them in community or environmental projects instills values of empathy and responsibility. Children raised with a global perspective grow into adults who value diversity and contribute to a more inclusive world.

The journey toward global connection is not without challenges. Miscommunication, cultural misunderstandings, and systemic inequalities require patience, humility, and persistence to overcome. However, the rewards—deeper understanding, enriched perspectives, and a shared sense of purpose—make these efforts profoundly worthwhile.

Ultimately, global connection is about recognizing that we are part of something greater than ourselves. It is an invitation to step beyond individualism and embrace a collective vision of well-being and harmony. By fostering compassion, collaboration, and accountability, we contribute to a world where diversity is celebrated, challenges are shared, and solutions are co-created.

Through global connection, we honor the truth that humanity is one family, united by shared dreams, challenges, and aspirations. In this unity, we find strength, purpose, and the hope of a brighter future—one shaped by empathy, cooperation, and a deep reverence for the interconnected web of life.

Chapter 27
Awakening Consciousness

The awakening of consciousness is a transformative process that invites individuals to step beyond the confines of conditioned thought and into a state of expanded awareness. It is the recognition of one's interconnectedness with all life, a shift in perspective that reveals the deeper truths of existence. Awakening consciousness is not a singular event but an ongoing journey, a practice of living with intention, clarity, and alignment.

At the heart of awakening is the realization that there is more to life than the physical and material. It begins with a sense of curiosity or restlessness, a feeling that something is missing despite outward success or fulfillment. This inner stirring is often the first sign of a deeper awakening, prompting questions such as: *Who am I? Why am I here? What is the nature of reality?* These questions mark the beginning of a journey inward.

The process of awakening often unfolds in stages. The first stage is awareness, where individuals become conscious of their thoughts, emotions, and patterns. They begin to question the beliefs and assumptions that have shaped their reality, uncovering the unconscious programming that influences their choices. Practices like mindfulness, meditation, and journaling provide tools for this self-reflection, creating space for greater clarity and insight.

The next stage is deconstruction, a period of letting go. As individuals examine their conditioned beliefs, they often find that many no longer serve their highest good. This can be a challenging phase, as it involves releasing attachments to old identities, roles, or ways of being. However, it is also liberating, creating room for new perspectives and possibilities to emerge.

During awakening, many individuals experience heightened sensitivity to energy and emotion. They may become more attuned to the needs of their bodies, the emotions of others, or the vibrational quality of their environment. While this sensitivity can feel overwhelming, it is also a gift, offering a deeper connection to the present moment and the flow of life.

A significant aspect of awakening is the recognition of interconnectedness. As consciousness expands, individuals begin to see themselves not as separate beings but as part of a larger whole. This realization fosters compassion, empathy, and a sense of responsibility for the well-being of others and the planet. It also dissolves the illusion of separation, creating a profound sense of unity and belonging.

Awakening consciousness often involves moments of profound insight or epiphany. These "aha" moments may arise during meditation, in nature, or even in the midst of ordinary life. They offer glimpses of a greater reality, moments of clarity that shift perspectives and inspire transformation. While these experiences are fleeting, they leave lasting impressions, serving as guideposts on the journey.

Shadow work is a crucial part of awakening, as it involves confronting and integrating the aspects of the self that have been hidden or suppressed. The shadow holds the fears, insecurities, and wounds that we often avoid facing. By bringing these aspects into awareness with compassion, individuals reclaim their wholeness and unlock deeper levels of authenticity and freedom.

The role of intuition becomes central during awakening. Intuition is the inner knowing that arises beyond logic or reason, a direct connection to the wisdom of the soul. As individuals awaken, they learn to trust this inner guidance, using it to navigate life's complexities with clarity and confidence. Practices like meditation, energy work, or spending time in nature strengthen this intuitive connection.

Awakening also involves a shift in values. As consciousness expands, priorities often change, moving away from material pursuits and toward experiences that nourish the soul. Simplicity, authenticity, and connection take precedence, reflecting a deeper alignment with one's true essence. This shift brings greater fulfillment, as actions and choices are rooted in meaning and purpose.

The experience of awakening is not without challenges. Letting go of old identities and beliefs can feel destabilizing, and the journey may include moments of doubt, fear, or confusion. However, these challenges are also opportunities for growth, as they prompt individuals to deepen their trust in the process and their connection to the greater whole.

Spiritual practices play a vital role in awakening consciousness. Meditation creates a space for stillness and self-awareness, while yoga harmonizes body, mind, and spirit. Breathwork clears energetic blockages, and journaling provides a means to explore and integrate insights. These practices serve as anchors, supporting individuals through the transitions of awakening.

The journey of awakening is deeply personal, yet it also connects individuals to a collective process. As more people awaken, they contribute to a shift in global consciousness, fostering greater empathy, collaboration, and a sense of shared purpose. This collective awakening holds the potential to address the challenges of our time, from environmental degradation to social inequality, with wisdom and compassion.

For those seeking to awaken consciousness, the journey begins with a willingness to explore. Curiosity, openness, and the courage to question are the seeds of transformation. Engaging with spiritual teachings, reading about others' journeys, or seeking guidance from mentors or communities can provide inspiration and support.

Awakening is not about escaping the world but engaging with it more fully. It is about bringing higher awareness into everyday life, from the way we interact with others to the choices we make. It is a call to live authentically, to align actions with values, and to contribute positively to the world.

Stories of awakening illustrate the transformative power of this process. An individual trapped in the monotony of routine discovers a passion for art, awakening their creativity and sense of purpose. A person grieving a loss finds solace in meditation, connecting with a sense of unity and eternal presence. A professional seeking success reevaluates their priorities, shifting toward a life of simplicity and meaning.

Ultimately, awakening consciousness is a journey home to the self. It is the realization that we are not separate from the universe but expressions of its infinite creativity and love. This awareness brings freedom, peace, and a profound sense of belonging, transforming not only the individual but also the world they inhabit.

The awakening of consciousness invites us to see with new eyes, to live with open hearts, and to embrace the boundless potential within and around us. It is a journey of remembering who we are and why we are here, a process of becoming fully alive, fully present, and fully connected to the wonder of existence.

Chapter 28
Harmony in Spaces

The spaces we inhabit hold a profound influence over our well-being, energy, and state of mind. From our homes to our workplaces, the arrangement, energy, and aesthetics of these environments can either uplift and inspire us or drain and stagnate us. Achieving harmony in spaces is a core principle of holistic living, one that recognizes that our surroundings are a reflection of our inner world. By cultivating intentional, balanced environments, we create sanctuaries that nurture the body, mind, and spirit.

At the foundation of harmonious spaces is the concept of energy flow. Ancient practices like Feng Shui and Vastu Shastra emphasize that the energy, or *chi*, in a space must flow freely to promote health, happiness, and prosperity. Blockages in this energy—caused by clutter, disrepair, or poor arrangement—can lead to feelings of stress, fatigue, or stagnation. Conversely, a space with clear, intentional energy fosters clarity, vitality, and creativity.

The first step in creating harmony in spaces is decluttering. Removing items that no longer serve a purpose or bring joy clears both physical and energetic space. Clutter not only occupies room but also creates mental noise, making it harder to focus and relax. By letting go of excess, we create an environment that feels open, serene, and supportive of our goals and intentions.

The layout of a space also plays a crucial role in its energy. Furniture placement, lighting, and pathways should encourage a sense of flow and balance. For example, arranging seating to face natural light or a calming view promotes relaxation and positivity, while avoiding blocked doorways or overcrowded corners ensures the free movement of energy.

Colors and materials further influence the energy of a space. Earth tones like browns and greens evoke grounding and stability, while lighter hues like whites and pastels create a sense of openness and calm. Natural materials such as wood, stone, and cotton enhance the connection to nature, bringing warmth and authenticity to the environment. Choosing colors and textures that align with personal preferences and intentions creates a space that feels uniquely nurturing.

Lighting is another essential element of harmonious spaces. Natural light is ideal, as it regulates circadian rhythms, boosts mood, and enhances focus. For spaces with limited natural light, soft, warm lighting creates a welcoming atmosphere, while dimmers allow for flexibility depending on the time of day or activity. Candles, too, bring a gentle, soothing glow that promotes relaxation and introspection.

The inclusion of nature in a space, often referred to as biophilic design, enhances its harmony. Plants purify the air, reduce stress, and bring a sense of vitality and growth. From lush greenery in living rooms to small potted herbs in kitchens, the presence of plants fosters a deeper connection to the earth and its cycles. Incorporating elements like water features, natural wood, or even artwork depicting landscapes further strengthens this bond.

Creating harmony in spaces also involves engaging the senses. Aromatherapy, for example, uses essential oils like lavender, eucalyptus, or citrus to evoke feelings of calm, energy, or focus. Soft music, nature sounds, or silence sets the tone for different activities, whether work, meditation, or relaxation. Textures, from plush rugs to smooth stones, invite touch and add dimension to the environment. By mindfully incorporating sensory elements, we make spaces not only functional but also nourishing.

Each space in a home or workplace serves a distinct purpose, and its design should align with that intention. Bedrooms, for instance, are sanctuaries for rest and rejuvenation. Simple, soothing colors, minimal electronics, and comfortable bedding create an environment conducive to sleep and relaxation. Kitchens, as spaces for nourishment and gathering, benefit from warm, inviting designs and efficient organization. Workspaces, whether at home or in an office, thrive on order, natural light, and inspiring touches like art or personal items.

The energy of a space is also influenced by its history and occupants. Cleansing rituals, such as burning sage, Palo Santo, or incense, clear stagnant or negative energy and create a fresh, vibrant atmosphere. Intentionally setting the tone for a space—through affirmations, prayers, or gratitude practices—imbues it with positive energy and purpose.

Personalization is key to creating spaces that feel harmonious and authentic. While design trends can offer inspiration, the most meaningful spaces reflect individual tastes, values, and memories. Displaying photographs, keepsakes, or art that resonates with the heart transforms a house into a home and an office into a personal sanctuary.

Harmonizing shared spaces requires collaboration and consideration. Whether living with family, roommates, or partners, open communication about needs and preferences fosters mutual respect and understanding. Creating common areas that balance different styles and priorities ensures that everyone feels comfortable and represented.

The impact of harmonious spaces extends beyond the physical. A clutter-free, well-organized environment reduces stress, enhances focus, and supports mental clarity. Spaces that are intentionally designed for activities like meditation, yoga, or creative pursuits encourage deeper engagement and flow. Even small changes, like rearranging furniture or adding a plant, can shift the energy of a space and uplift the spirit.

Workplaces, too, benefit from harmonious design. Open, well-lit layouts promote collaboration and creativity, while designated quiet areas support focus and reflection. Incorporating elements like greenery, natural light, and ergonomic furniture fosters well-being, increasing both productivity and satisfaction.

Children's spaces hold particular significance in their development and well-being. Creating environments that inspire creativity, curiosity, and comfort helps children thrive. Organized, accessible storage encourages independence, while areas for play and exploration foster imagination and joy. Including children in the design process teaches them the value of harmony and personal expression.

Stories of transformation through harmonious spaces illustrate their profound impact. A person struggling with anxiety finds calm and focus after simplifying their living space and introducing calming colors and scents. A family strengthens their bond by creating a shared area for meals and conversations. A professional reclaims energy and creativity by decluttering their workspace and incorporating natural elements.

Ultimately, harmony in spaces reflects harmony within. By mindfully curating our environments, we create spaces that align with our values, support our intentions, and nurture our well-being. These spaces become more than places to live or work—they become sanctuaries that inspire and sustain us.

In embracing harmony in spaces, we honor the connection between our outer world and inner state. We transform our surroundings into reflections of who we are and who we aspire to be, creating environments that uplift, empower, and heal. Through these intentional choices, we not only design spaces—we design lives filled with beauty, balance, and purpose.

Chapter 29
Ancestral Practices

Ancestral practices are profound sources of wisdom, deeply rooted in the rhythms of nature and the understanding of life's interconnectedness. These traditions, passed down through generations, carry the knowledge of healing, spirituality, and community that sustained humanity long before modern science and technology. Reconnecting with these practices is not merely about honoring the past—it is about integrating timeless insights into contemporary life to foster balance, healing, and purpose.

At the core of ancestral practices lies a profound respect for the natural world. Indigenous cultures and ancient traditions often view nature not as a resource to be exploited but as a living system to be honored and harmonized with. The cycles of the moon, the movement of the seasons, and the elements of earth, water, fire, and air are woven into rituals and ceremonies, serving as reminders of humanity's place within the greater whole.

One of the most enduring aspects of ancestral wisdom is the use of natural medicine. Herbs, roots, and plants have been used for millennia to heal the body, mind, and spirit. Practices such as Ayurveda, Traditional Chinese Medicine (TCM), and shamanic healing emphasize the energetic and spiritual properties of natural remedies alongside their physical benefits. For example, turmeric is valued in Ayurveda for its anti-inflammatory properties, while sage is used in many Indigenous cultures for energetic cleansing and protection.

Rituals play a significant role in ancestral practices, serving as bridges between the physical and spiritual realms. These rituals often involve offerings, prayers, and symbolic acts that align individuals with the forces of nature and the divine. Fire ceremonies, for instance, are used to release the old and welcome the new, while water rituals symbolize purification and renewal. These acts are not mere formalities; they are opportunities for transformation and connection.

Ancestral practices also emphasize the power of storytelling. Oral traditions, myths, and legends preserve cultural identity and impart moral and spiritual lessons. These stories carry archetypal wisdom, resonating across time and cultures. They remind us of our shared humanity, offering guidance on how to navigate challenges, honor values, and live in harmony with others and the world.

Music and dance are integral to many ancestral practices, serving as expressions of emotion, celebration, and spiritual connection. Drumming, for example, is a universal practice found in cultures worldwide, used to alter states of consciousness, heal, and build community. Traditional dances often mimic the movements of nature—waves, animals, or the wind—reflecting the unity of life. These practices remind us of the healing power of rhythm and movement.

The concept of ancestral wisdom is not limited to cultural traditions; it also encompasses the knowledge held within our genetic and energetic lineage. Epigenetics, the study of how experiences and behaviors can influence gene expression, suggests that the trauma, resilience, and wisdom of our ancestors live on in us. Practices such as ancestral meditation or family constellations help individuals explore and heal inherited patterns, fostering a deeper connection to their lineage and identity.

Ancestor reverence is a common thread across many traditions. Honoring those who came before us acknowledges their contributions and sacrifices while seeking their guidance and protection. Altars dedicated to ancestors, offerings of food or flowers, and ceremonies of remembrance create a living bond between the past and present. These acts of reverence foster gratitude, grounding individuals in their heritage and providing a sense of belonging.

Ceremonial practices like sweat lodges, vision quests, and plant medicine journeys exemplify the depth of ancestral healing traditions. These experiences often involve entering altered states of consciousness to access higher wisdom, release trauma, or gain clarity. While these practices require preparation, guidance, and respect, they offer profound opportunities for transformation and spiritual awakening.

Ancestral practices also emphasize the importance of community and interdependence. Rituals and ceremonies are often collective experiences, bringing people together to celebrate, mourn, or seek guidance. This sense of shared purpose strengthens bonds, fosters empathy, and reminds individuals that they are part of something greater than themselves.

In the modern world, reconnecting with ancestral practices can feel like a return to the essence of life. Simple acts like growing herbs, cooking traditional recipes, or meditating in nature revive ancient wisdom in accessible ways. These practices serve as anchors, grounding individuals in the present while connecting them to the timeless.

Integrating ancestral practices into daily life requires respect and intentionality. It is essential to approach these traditions with humility, seeking to understand their origins and cultural significance. For those exploring practices outside their heritage, engaging with teachers, elders, or communities from those traditions fosters authenticity and avoids appropriation.

The revival of ancestral practices is also a form of resistance against cultural erasure and environmental destruction. Indigenous knowledge systems, for example, hold critical insights into sustainable living, biodiversity conservation, and climate resilience. Protecting and amplifying these voices honors their wisdom while addressing global challenges.

Teaching ancestral practices to children preserves this wisdom for future generations. Activities like storytelling, learning traditional crafts, or participating in family rituals instill values of respect, gratitude, and connection. These lessons provide children with a sense of identity and continuity, helping them navigate the complexities of modern life with rootedness and resilience.

Stories of transformation through ancestral practices highlight their enduring relevance. A person struggling with a sense of disconnection finds grounding through learning their cultural dances. An individual burdened by generational trauma discovers healing through ancestral meditation and forgiveness rituals. A community strengthens its bond by reviving traditional ceremonies that celebrate the seasons and honor the earth.

Ultimately, ancestral practices are pathways to remembering—remembering our connection to nature, to our lineage, and to the deeper truths of existence. They remind us that we are not separate from the world around us but part of a continuum that spans time and space.

By integrating ancestral practices into modern life, we honor the wisdom of those who came before us while creating a bridge to the future. These traditions, rich with meaning and insight, guide us toward a life of balance, harmony, and reverence for the interconnected web of life.

In embracing ancestral practices, we rediscover not only the wisdom of the past but also the essence of who we are. These practices ground us in our humanity, inspire us to live with purpose, and connect us to the timeless rhythm of life—a rhythm that continues to pulse through us and the generations to come.

Chapter 30
Life Purpose

Finding and living one's life purpose is a journey of self-discovery and alignment, a process of uncovering the unique contribution one is meant to offer to the world. Purpose provides a sense of direction and fulfillment, transforming ordinary existence into a meaningful adventure. While the search for purpose may feel elusive or overwhelming, it is ultimately about connecting with one's essence and translating that connection into action.

At its core, life purpose is not necessarily about grand achievements or recognition but about authenticity. It is the expression of one's deepest values, talents, and passions in a way that serves both the self and the greater whole. Purpose aligns the heart, mind, and spirit, creating a sense of harmony and flow in daily life.

The journey toward discovering purpose often begins with introspection. Questions like *What brings me joy? What do I care about deeply? How can I make a difference?* serve as guideposts, helping individuals uncover their unique path. Practices such as journaling, meditation, or vision-boarding offer tools for exploring these questions, revealing patterns and insights that point toward purpose.

For many, purpose is tied to their natural talents or interests. These are the activities that come easily, the skills that feel intuitive, or the passions that ignite enthusiasm. Reflecting on what others have admired or sought help for can also provide clues. A person who is naturally empathetic, for example, may find purpose in caregiving, counseling, or advocacy.

Passion alone, however, is not the sole determinant of purpose. Purpose often lies at the intersection of passion, skills, and service to others. The Japanese concept of *ikigai*, which translates to "reason for being," illustrates this beautifully. It encourages individuals to find the overlap between what they love, what they are good at, what the world needs, and what they can be rewarded for.

Living a purposeful life does not necessarily require radical change. Purpose can be infused into existing roles and routines. A teacher may find purpose in inspiring students to think critically, a parent in nurturing future generations, or an artist in evoking emotions through their work. Purpose is not limited to professional endeavors—it can also be found in personal relationships, community involvement, or spiritual growth.

Challenges often play a role in shaping one's purpose. Adversity, pain, or setbacks can serve as catalysts for transformation, revealing strengths and perspectives that lead to meaningful contributions. For instance, someone who has overcome illness may feel called to support others on their healing journeys. Rather than viewing difficulties as barriers, the holistic perspective sees them as opportunities for growth and alignment.

Purpose is also dynamic, evolving with life's seasons and experiences. What feels purposeful in youth may differ from what resonates in later years. This evolution is natural and reflects the unfolding of one's inner and outer worlds. Staying open to change and reevaluating priorities ensures that purpose remains authentic and aligned.

The pursuit of purpose often requires stepping outside one's comfort zone. Taking risks, trying new activities, or embracing uncertainty are part of the process. While fear or doubt may arise, purpose provides the courage to move forward. It reminds individuals that growth lies on the other side of challenge, and that each step, no matter how small, contributes to the larger journey.

Community plays an important role in supporting purpose. Surrounding oneself with like-minded individuals or mentors who encourage exploration and growth fosters inspiration and accountability. Engaging with communities that share similar values or goals provides a sense of belonging and amplifies the impact of purposeful actions.

Spiritual practices offer guidance on the path to purpose. Meditation, prayer, or energy work connect individuals to their higher selves and the universal flow of life, providing clarity and inspiration. These practices remind individuals that purpose is not only personal but also connected to something greater—whether it be humanity, nature, or the divine.

Purpose is not always about doing; it is also about being. Living with purpose means showing up authentically, regardless of external circumstances. It involves embodying values such as kindness, integrity, or curiosity in everyday interactions. These small, consistent acts of alignment create a ripple effect, positively influencing others and the world.

Gratitude enhances the experience of purpose. By appreciating what is already meaningful in one's life, individuals deepen their connection to purpose. Gratitude also shifts focus from lack to abundance, fostering a sense of fulfillment and motivation. Reflecting on moments of joy, connection, or contribution illuminates the threads of purpose already woven into life.

For children, fostering a sense of purpose begins with encouragement and exploration. Allowing them to pursue interests, ask questions, and express themselves freely nurtures their natural curiosity and creativity. Teaching them the value of contribution—whether through acts of kindness, teamwork, or responsibility—lays the foundation for purposeful living.

Stories of purpose inspire and affirm its power. A person who transforms a love for gardening into a community program that feeds the hungry. An entrepreneur who builds a sustainable business that aligns with their values. A retiree who discovers new purpose by mentoring young professionals. These examples remind us that purpose can be found and expressed in countless ways.

Living with purpose brings profound benefits. It fosters resilience, providing a sense of meaning even in the face of adversity. It enhances well-being, as actions feel aligned and fulfilling. It strengthens relationships, as authenticity deepens connections. Perhaps most importantly, it creates a sense of legacy, as purposeful actions leave a positive imprint on the world.

For those who feel uncertain about their purpose, the key is to begin with curiosity and action. Purpose often reveals itself not through thinking but through doing. Volunteering, learning new skills, or simply pursuing what feels meaningful in the moment creates momentum, allowing purpose to unfold naturally.

Ultimately, life purpose is not a destination but a journey. It is not about finding a single, fixed answer but about living with intention and alignment. It is about showing up fully, embracing both challenges and joys, and contributing one's unique essence to the world.

In discovering and living their purpose, individuals align with their highest potential, creating lives of meaning, connection, and fulfillment. Through this alignment, they not only transform themselves but also inspire and uplift those around them.

Life purpose is a gift, an invitation to live authentically and make a difference. By embracing it, we honor our unique place in the tapestry of existence, contributing to the beauty and harmony of the greater whole.

Chapter 31
Holistic Spirituality in Childhood

Introducing children to holistic spirituality is one of the most meaningful ways to nurture empathy, resilience, and a sense of connection to the world around them. Unlike traditional religious frameworks, holistic spirituality focuses on universal values such as kindness, mindfulness, and interconnection, helping children grow into thoughtful, balanced, and compassionate individuals. This chapter explores how holistic practices can be adapted to children's developmental stages, fostering their emotional and spiritual well-being from an early age.

Children are naturally attuned to wonder and curiosity, qualities that lie at the heart of holistic spirituality. They observe the world with fresh eyes, marveling at the simple beauty of nature, the mystery of the universe, and the joy of discovery. Cultivating this innate sense of awe helps children develop a spiritual foundation that will serve them throughout their lives.

One of the most accessible ways to introduce holistic spirituality is through mindfulness. Practices such as breathing exercises, sensory awareness, or quiet reflection teach children to center themselves and connect with the present moment. Mindfulness activities can be playful and engaging, such as observing the movement of a feather in the air or listening to the sound of rain. These practices help children manage stress, regulate emotions, and develop focus.

Gratitude is another cornerstone of holistic spirituality for children. Encouraging them to express gratitude for simple joys—a favorite toy, a sunny day, or time with family—instills a habit of appreciation. Creating a family gratitude practice, such as sharing one thing each person is thankful for at dinner, fosters a positive and connected atmosphere. Gratitude journals designed for children, with prompts and creative spaces for drawings, make this practice both fun and meaningful.

Connection to nature plays a vital role in a child's spiritual development. Activities like planting a garden, observing wildlife, or collecting leaves deepen their understanding of life's cycles and interdependence. Time spent in natural settings also nurtures a sense of calm and clarity, grounding children in the rhythms of the earth. For younger children, storytelling about the natural world—such as tales of the moon, stars, or animals—bridges imagination and connection.

Creativity is another powerful avenue for exploring spirituality. Art, music, and storytelling allow children to express their inner worlds and explore ideas of meaning, beauty, and connection. Painting a picture of their "happy place" or writing a story about a kind act helps them articulate their feelings and values. These activities encourage self-expression while deepening their sense of purpose and connection.

Rituals tailored to children bring structure and significance to their spiritual experiences. Simple practices, such as lighting a candle during quiet time, saying a short blessing before meals, or celebrating the changing seasons, create moments of reflection and intention. These rituals provide a sense of continuity and grounding, helping children feel connected to something larger than themselves.

Teaching empathy is central to holistic spirituality. Activities that foster kindness and understanding, such as volunteering, helping a friend, or making a gift for someone in need, encourage children to consider others' feelings and perspectives. Reading stories that highlight themes of compassion and fairness further reinforces these values, showing children how their actions can positively impact the world.

Movement and physical practices like yoga are excellent ways to engage children in holistic spirituality. Yoga for kids incorporates simple poses, games, and breathing techniques that promote physical awareness, balance, and calm. These practices also help children feel more in tune with their bodies, building a sense of self-trust and inner strength.

Mindful communication nurtures a child's spiritual awareness by encouraging them to articulate their feelings and listen to others with openness and respect. Family discussions that emphasize active listening, nonjudgmental responses, and curiosity create a safe space for children to express themselves. This habit of mindful communication strengthens relationships and fosters emotional intelligence.

For parents and caregivers, modeling holistic spirituality is one of the most impactful ways to inspire children. Children learn by observing, so practicing mindfulness, expressing gratitude, or demonstrating kindness in daily life sets a powerful example. Sharing personal practices, such as journaling or meditating, provides children with tangible tools they can adopt as they grow.

Holistic spirituality for children also includes the exploration of values like respect for diversity and unity. Celebrating cultural traditions, exploring world myths, and learning about different beliefs teach children to appreciate the richness of human experience. This broader perspective helps them understand that while people may have unique ways of expressing spirituality, the core values of love, respect, and connection are universal.

Challenges often arise in helping children navigate their emotions and spiritual growth. It is essential to meet children where they are, offering practices that align with their age and temperament. Encouraging questions and discussions about life, death, or purpose helps them explore their inner thoughts without fear or judgment. Providing reassurance and creating a safe environment allows children to develop their spiritual identity at their own pace.

As children grow, their understanding of spirituality deepens. Adolescents, for example, may gravitate toward practices like journaling, meditation, or exploring philosophical ideas. Supporting their evolving interests and encouraging open dialogue fosters a sense of trust and mutual respect. Parents and caregivers can continue to serve as guides, offering wisdom while honoring the child's autonomy.

Stories of children engaging with holistic spirituality highlight its transformative impact. A shy child gains confidence and calm through a daily mindfulness routine. A family grows closer by sharing gratitude practices and exploring nature together. A young artist discovers a sense of purpose by expressing their values through drawing and painting. These moments demonstrate how spirituality, when nurtured holistically, becomes a lifelong source of strength and inspiration.

Ultimately, introducing holistic spirituality to children is an act of love and empowerment. It provides them with tools to navigate life's challenges, connect with others, and find meaning in their experiences. It instills values that will guide them throughout their lives, helping them grow into compassionate, balanced, and self-aware individuals.

Holistic spirituality reminds children—and adults—that they are part of something greater, a vast and interconnected web of life. By nurturing this awareness, we help them build a foundation of purpose, peace, and connection, inspiring them to contribute positively to the world. Through this journey, children learn not only to thrive but to live with intention, gratitude, and love.

Chapter 32
Energetic Communication

Communication is more than the exchange of words; it is an energetic interplay that shapes relationships, emotions, and understanding. Energetic communication acknowledges the unseen currents that flow between individuals, including body language, tone, intent, and vibrational resonance. By cultivating awareness of this dynamic, we can enhance the clarity, empathy, and authenticity of our interactions, fostering deeper and more meaningful connections.

At its foundation, energetic communication begins with presence. Being fully present in a conversation allows us to truly hear and feel the other person, beyond the words they speak. Presence is about setting aside distractions and giving undivided attention, creating a space where both individuals feel valued and understood. This attentiveness conveys respect and care, forming the basis for authentic communication.

The energy we bring to a conversation often determines its tone and outcome. Approaching interactions with calmness, openness, and genuine curiosity creates an inviting atmosphere, encouraging others to share freely. Conversely, entering a conversation with judgment, defensiveness, or agitation can block connection and understanding. Cultivating self-awareness of our emotional state and energy before engaging with others helps set a constructive tone.

Body language is a powerful form of energetic communication. Gestures, facial expressions, and posture often convey more than words alone. For example, an open stance, steady eye contact, and relaxed shoulders signal attentiveness and approachability. Conversely, crossed arms, avoidance of eye contact, or tense movements may indicate discomfort or disinterest. Becoming attuned to our own body language and that of others enhances mutual understanding and emotional resonance.

Tone of voice is another essential element of energetic communication. The way something is said—its pitch, pace, and volume—can amplify or diminish its impact. A gentle, steady tone often conveys care and sincerity, while a rushed or abrupt tone may create tension or misunderstanding. Mindful use of tone helps ensure that our spoken words align with the energy we wish to convey.

Listening is at the heart of energetic communication. Active listening involves more than hearing words; it requires tuning into the speaker's emotional energy and underlying message. Pausing before responding, asking thoughtful questions, and reflecting on what has been said demonstrate that we are fully engaged. This depth of listening creates a sense of safety and validation, fostering trust and connection.

Empathy is the bridge that connects our energy to that of others. It involves stepping into another's perspective, feeling with them rather than for them. Empathy does not require fixing or solving someone else's problems but simply being present with their emotions. Energetically, empathy is about holding space—a practice that conveys understanding and compassion without judgment or expectation.

Intent is a subtle but profound aspect of energetic communication. The energy behind our words often carries more weight than the words themselves. For instance, offering advice with genuine care and humility resonates differently than doing so with a desire to control or criticize. Checking our intentions before speaking ensures that our communication aligns with our values and promotes connection rather than division.

Boundaries are a crucial component of energetic communication. While openness is essential, so is the ability to protect our energy and respect the boundaries of others. Clear, assertive communication about needs and limits prevents misunderstandings and fosters mutual respect. For example, expressing a need for personal space or time to process emotions helps maintain balance and authenticity in relationships.

Nonverbal energy exchange often occurs unconsciously but can be a powerful tool when used intentionally. Practices like offering a warm smile, a comforting touch, or even maintaining a peaceful presence can convey support and understanding without words. These gestures create a field of positive energy that others naturally respond to, enhancing the quality of connection.

Mindfulness is key to mastering energetic communication. By staying present with our thoughts, emotions, and reactions, we become more aware of how our energy affects others and vice versa. Practices like breathwork or brief pauses during conversations help reset our energy, ensuring that we respond rather than react. This mindfulness transforms communication into a deliberate and meaningful exchange.

Energetic communication also extends to how we communicate with ourselves. The inner dialogue we maintain shapes not only our relationship with ourselves but also the energy we bring into interactions with others. Practicing self-compassion, affirmations, and honest reflection creates a balanced and positive internal energy, which radiates outward.

Cultural and personal differences can influence energetic communication, highlighting the importance of adaptability and sensitivity. Being open to learning about others' communication styles—whether influenced by cultural norms, personality types, or life experiences—enhances mutual understanding. This flexibility creates a bridge across differences, fostering inclusivity and respect.

Energy can also linger in spaces, influencing the tone of communication. For example, an uncluttered, welcoming room with natural light and soothing colors fosters calm and openness, while a chaotic or harsh environment may breed tension. Setting the stage for communication—whether through clearing the space, lighting a candle, or simply creating a quiet moment—helps align the energy for constructive interaction.

Conflict is an inevitable part of communication, but energetic awareness can transform how it unfolds. Approaching disagreements with calm energy and an intention to understand rather than win shifts the dynamic from confrontation to collaboration. Techniques like paraphrasing the other person's points, taking pauses, and focusing on shared goals help resolve conflicts constructively.

Children offer profound lessons in energetic communication. They are often more attuned to nonverbal energy than adults and respond deeply to authenticity and presence. Communicating with children involves simplicity, patience, and an open heart, emphasizing the energy behind the words more than their complexity. Modeling positive communication habits teaches children to express themselves honestly and empathetically.

Stories of transformation through energetic communication highlight its potential to deepen relationships. A couple struggling with misunderstanding strengthens their bond by practicing active listening and setting aside judgment. A team leader fosters harmony and collaboration in the workplace by addressing conflict with empathy and clear intent. A parent rebuilds trust with their child by embracing mindful communication and emotional openness.

Ultimately, energetic communication is about alignment—ensuring that what we say, how we say it, and the energy we project are congruent. It is about connecting authentically, respecting boundaries, and creating spaces for mutual understanding and growth.

By mastering the art of energetic communication, we transform not only our relationships but also our connection to the world. This practice nurtures deeper empathy, authenticity, and harmony, enabling us to express ourselves fully while honoring the energy of others. Through this alignment, communication becomes not just an exchange of information but a profound and transformative act of connection.

Chapter 33
Balancing Masculine and Feminine Energies

Within each of us exists a dynamic interplay of masculine and feminine energies, regardless of gender. These energies are not tied to societal roles or stereotypes but represent universal principles that shape how we think, feel, and act. Masculine energy embodies qualities like action, logic, and structure, while feminine energy encompasses intuition, creativity, and receptivity. Achieving balance between these energies is essential for living a harmonious and fulfilling life.

Understanding the essence of these energies is the first step toward integration. The masculine is often described as the energy of doing—it is linear, goal-oriented, and focused on action and achievement. It represents the drive to create, protect, and provide. The feminine, on the other hand, is the energy of being—it is cyclical, fluid, and nurturing. It reflects the capacity to receive, feel, and connect deeply with oneself and others.

In a balanced state, masculine and feminine energies complement and enhance one another. The masculine provides direction and structure to the feminine's flow and creativity, while the feminine softens and enriches the masculine's focus and drive. Together, they form a harmonious whole, enabling individuals to navigate life with both strength and grace.

Imbalances in these energies can lead to challenges. An overemphasis on masculine energy may result in rigidity, burnout, or disconnection from emotions, while an excess of feminine energy can manifest as passivity, indecision, or overwhelm. Recognizing these imbalances is the first step in restoring harmony, allowing each energy to express itself in a healthy and supportive way.

The journey toward balance begins with self-awareness. By observing how we approach challenges, relationships, and personal goals, we can identify which energy tends to dominate and where we might benefit from integrating its counterpart. Practices like journaling or mindfulness meditation help cultivate this awareness, offering insights into our energetic patterns and needs.

To cultivate masculine energy, individuals can focus on practices that build discipline, focus, and action. Setting clear goals, creating routines, or engaging in physical activities like strength training foster a sense of structure and purpose. Visualization and affirmations centered on confidence and determination amplify the masculine energy of forward momentum.

To nurture feminine energy, practices that encourage intuition, creativity, and flow are key. Activities like journaling, dancing, or spending time in nature connect individuals to their inner worlds and the rhythms of life. Allowing time for rest, play, and reflection honors the feminine energy of receptivity and renewal. Meditation, especially focused on the heart chakra, strengthens the feminine qualities of compassion and connection.

Relationships often provide a mirror for masculine and feminine dynamics. Healthy relationships involve a fluid exchange of these energies, with partners supporting and balancing one another. For instance, one partner may take on a nurturing role while the other provides structure, but these roles can and should shift as needed. Open communication and mutual respect ensure that neither energy dominates, fostering harmony and growth.

In the workplace, balancing masculine and feminine energies creates a dynamic and effective environment. Masculine energy drives productivity, decision-making, and goal-setting, while feminine energy enhances collaboration, creativity, and emotional intelligence. Leaders who integrate both energies are more adaptable and compassionate, inspiring trust and innovation within their teams.

The integration of these energies also supports emotional resilience. Masculine energy provides the strength to face challenges and take decisive action, while feminine energy allows for the processing and release of emotions. Together, they create a foundation for navigating adversity with both courage and sensitivity.

Cultural and societal influences often shape how individuals express masculine and feminine energies. Historically, many cultures have favored one energy over the other, creating imbalances in personal and collective dynamics. For example, an overemphasis on masculine traits like competition and dominance can lead to disconnection from the nurturing and collaborative qualities of the feminine. Recognizing and addressing these cultural patterns is an essential step toward holistic balance.

Healing the relationship between these energies often involves addressing internalized beliefs and wounds. For many, past experiences may have led to the suppression of one energy. For instance, someone raised to prioritize logic and achievement may struggle to embrace their emotions or creativity. Shadow work and inner child healing can uncover these blocks, allowing individuals to reclaim their full energetic expression.

Spiritual practices provide a pathway to integrating masculine and feminine energies. Yoga, for example, balances strength and flexibility, action and surrender. Breathwork harmonizes the active and receptive forces within the body, creating a sense of inner equilibrium. Energy healing practices like Reiki or chakra alignment specifically address imbalances in these energies, fostering harmony on a vibrational level.

The balance of masculine and feminine energies is also reflected in nature. The sun, with its steady, radiant energy, embodies the masculine, while the moon, with its cycles and changing phases, symbolizes the feminine. Observing and aligning with these natural rhythms reminds us of the importance of both energies in creating balance and flow.

Parenting offers a profound opportunity to model and nurture balanced energies. Encouraging children to express both their assertive and nurturing sides helps them grow into well-rounded individuals. For example, teaching a child to set boundaries (a masculine quality) while also valuing empathy and collaboration (feminine traits) creates a foundation for emotional intelligence and resilience.

Stories of transformation through balancing these energies reveal the profound impact of integration. A professional driven by masculine energy finds renewal and creativity by embracing feminine practices like mindfulness and self-care. An artist reconnects with their masculine energy, building the discipline and focus needed to bring their vision to life. A couple deepens their bond by exploring and harmonizing their energetic dynamics, creating a partnership rooted in mutual growth.

Ultimately, the balance of masculine and feminine energies is not about equality in every moment but about honoring what is needed in each situation. Sometimes, action and structure are required; other times, intuition and receptivity are the answer. By cultivating both energies, individuals gain the flexibility and wisdom to navigate life's complexities with grace and strength.

In embracing this balance, we connect with the full spectrum of our potential. We become more creative, compassionate, and focused, able to adapt to challenges and opportunities with ease. This integration fosters inner harmony, enriching not only our personal lives but also our relationships and contributions to the world.

The dance of masculine and feminine energies is an eternal rhythm, one that mirrors the balance of the universe itself. By honoring and harmonizing these forces within us, we align with the natural flow of life, creating a path of authenticity, connection, and fulfillment.

Chapter 34
Spiritual Reconnection

Spiritual reconnection is the process of returning to the essence of who we are and our relationship with the greater whole—whether that be the universe, nature, or the divine. In a world often consumed by busyness, material pursuits, and disconnection, this reconnection becomes a sacred act of remembering and renewal. It involves quieting the noise of the external world to hear the whispers of the soul and rekindling the sense of wonder and purpose that resides within.

Reconnection begins with intention. It is a conscious choice to seek alignment, to explore deeper truths, and to cultivate a relationship with the sacred. This intention opens the door to practices and experiences that nourish the spirit, providing a sense of grounding and transcendence. Whether one's spirituality is rooted in religion, nature, or personal exploration, the act of reconnection invites authenticity and presence.

One of the most profound ways to reconnect spiritually is through nature. The natural world is a living embodiment of balance, beauty, and interconnectedness. Spending time in nature—whether walking in the woods, sitting by a river, or gazing at the stars—creates space for reflection and awe. These moments remind us of our place within the larger tapestry of life, awakening a sense of unity and reverence.

Meditation serves as a cornerstone practice for spiritual reconnection. By quieting the mind and focusing on the breath or a mantra, individuals create a space to access their inner wisdom and connect with the divine. Meditation need not be complicated; even a few minutes of stillness each day can foster clarity, peace, and a sense of connection to something greater. Guided meditations, particularly those focused on themes like gratitude, compassion, or universal love, further deepen this practice.

Prayer, in its many forms, is another powerful tool for reconnection. Prayer can be formal or informal, spoken or silent, structured or spontaneous. It is less about the words themselves and more about the intention and openness behind them. Whether giving thanks, seeking guidance, or expressing longing, prayer creates a bridge between the individual and the divine, fostering a sense of communion and trust.

Rituals provide structure and meaning to the process of spiritual reconnection. Lighting a candle, setting an altar, or creating a daily gratitude practice transforms ordinary moments into sacred ones. Seasonal rituals, such as celebrating solstices, harvests, or new moons, align individuals with natural rhythms and cycles, deepening their connection to the flow of life.

Journaling offers a way to explore and articulate the spiritual journey. Writing about thoughts, emotions, or experiences provides clarity and insight, uncovering patterns and truths that might otherwise remain hidden. Prompts like "What brings me a sense of peace?" or "When do I feel most connected to the divine?" encourage reflection and foster a deeper understanding of one's spiritual path.

Music and sound play a unique role in spiritual reconnection. Sacred music, chanting, or instruments like singing bowls and gongs resonate with the body's energy, creating vibrations that calm the mind and elevate the spirit. Singing, humming, or simply listening to sounds that evoke peace and joy can open the heart and align one's energy with the sacred.

Spiritual reconnection often involves revisiting and healing the past. Unresolved emotions, regrets, or traumas can create barriers to connection, clouding the heart and mind. Practices like forgiveness, shadow work, or energy clearing help release these burdens, creating space for renewal and growth. By letting go of what no longer serves, individuals make room for deeper connection and understanding.

Community can also play a vital role in spiritual reconnection. Gathering with others for shared practices, such as meditation groups, spiritual circles, or religious services, fosters a sense of belonging and collective energy. The support and wisdom of a community often amplify individual efforts, reminding participants that they are not alone on their journey.

Sacred texts and teachings provide inspiration and guidance for those seeking reconnection. Whether drawn from religious traditions, philosophical works, or contemporary spiritual writings, these texts offer insights that resonate across time and cultures. Reading and reflecting on these teachings deepens understanding and provides tools for navigating the spiritual path.

Acts of service are another profound way to reconnect spiritually. Helping others, whether through volunteer work, small acts of kindness, or simply offering a listening ear, fosters a sense of purpose and connection. Service reminds us of our interconnectedness and reinforces the values of compassion and gratitude.

Spiritual reconnection is not always about profound experiences or dramatic realizations; it often lies in the small, everyday moments. A deep breath taken during a busy day, a silent moment of appreciation for a sunset, or the feeling of connection during a heartfelt conversation can all be acts of reconnection. These moments remind us that the sacred is always present, waiting to be acknowledged.

Challenges often arise on the path to spiritual reconnection. Doubt, fear, or feelings of unworthiness can create obstacles. However, these challenges are also opportunities for growth and transformation. By approaching them with curiosity and compassion, individuals deepen their understanding and strengthen their connection to the divine.

Children can teach us much about spiritual reconnection. Their natural sense of wonder, curiosity, and presence embodies qualities that are central to spirituality. Observing and engaging with children in activities like exploring nature, storytelling, or creating rituals rekindles these qualities in adults, offering a fresh perspective on the sacred.

Stories of transformation through spiritual reconnection highlight its profound impact. A person feeling lost and disconnected finds renewal through daily meditation and time spent in nature. An individual burdened by guilt experiences healing and peace through forgiveness rituals and prayer. A group of friends deepens their bond and collective purpose by creating a shared gratitude practice.

Ultimately, spiritual reconnection is about remembering—remembering our true essence, our connection to the greater whole, and the sacredness of life. It is a journey of returning home to ourselves and the universe, guided by love, curiosity, and trust.

In the act of spiritual reconnection, we awaken to the beauty, mystery, and interconnectedness of existence. We find not only peace and purpose but also a sense of belonging that transcends the individual self. This journey invites us to live with greater awareness, gratitude, and alignment, transforming both our inner and outer worlds.

Chapter 35
Transcendence of the Ego

The transcendence of the ego is one of the most profound steps on the path to holistic living and spiritual growth. The ego, often misunderstood as a purely negative force, is the part of the self that forms identity and separates us from others. It is concerned with survival, validation, and control, shaping much of how we interact with the world. While the ego serves an important role, its dominance can lead to conflict, insecurity, and disconnection from deeper truths. Transcending the ego does not mean eliminating it but rather placing it in balance, allowing us to live with greater freedom, authenticity, and unity.

The ego creates the illusion of separation, encouraging us to see ourselves as distinct from others and the world around us. This perspective fosters competition, comparison, and attachment to external achievements or possessions. The first step in transcending the ego is recognizing its influence—becoming aware of the thoughts, behaviors, and reactions that stem from egoic patterns. This awareness is not about judgment but observation, creating space for reflection and growth.

Ego-driven living often revolves around fear and desire. Fear of failure, rejection, or loss drives us to protect and defend the self, while desires for recognition, power, or material wealth seek to affirm our worth. These patterns keep us in a cycle of striving and resistance, disconnecting us from the present moment and the deeper aspects of our being. Transcending the ego requires shifting our focus from fear and desire to trust and acceptance, embracing life as it unfolds.

Mindfulness is a powerful tool for transcending the ego. By observing our thoughts and emotions without attachment, we begin to see the ego's patterns more clearly. Practices like meditation, breathwork, or simply pausing to reflect during moments of reactivity help us detach from the ego's grip and connect with the stillness of our true self. This practice builds a foundation of inner peace and clarity.

Another key aspect of ego transcendence is surrender. The ego thrives on control—on the need to shape outcomes, prove itself, or hold onto identities. Surrendering does not mean giving up but releasing the need for control and trusting the flow of life. This act of letting go allows us to align with the natural rhythms of existence, freeing us from unnecessary struggle and resistance.

Humility is an antidote to the ego's dominance. It involves recognizing that we are part of a greater whole, not separate or superior to others. Humility fosters a sense of interconnectedness, encouraging collaboration, empathy, and respect. Practices like gratitude, service, and acknowledging the contributions of others nurture humility and soften the ego's need for validation.

The concept of the "observer self" or higher self is central to ego transcendence. This is the part of us that witnesses our thoughts, emotions, and actions without attachment or judgment. By cultivating this awareness, we can step back from the ego's narratives and recognize them as temporary constructs rather than absolute truths. This shift empowers us to respond to life with wisdom and intention rather than react out of habit or fear.

Shadow work is another transformative practice on the path to transcending the ego. The shadow represents the parts of ourselves that we suppress or deny, often because they conflict with the ego's desired image. By exploring and integrating these aspects with compassion, we release the energy spent on repression and become more whole. This integration reduces the ego's grip, allowing us to live with greater authenticity and balance.

Forgiveness plays a vital role in ego transcendence. The ego clings to grievances, using them to justify feelings of separation, victimhood, or superiority. Forgiveness, both of ourselves and others, dissolves these barriers, creating space for healing and connection. It is not about condoning harm but about freeing ourselves from the weight of resentment and the stories the ego creates around it.

The practice of detachment is also essential. The ego often identifies with roles, possessions, or achievements, equating them with self-worth. Detachment does not mean rejecting these things but recognizing that they do not define us. By releasing attachment, we find freedom and discover our true essence, which is independent of external circumstances.

Transcending the ego also involves cultivating a sense of purpose beyond the self. When we align our actions with values such as compassion, service, or creativity, we transcend the ego's need for personal gain and connect with a higher vision. This shift fosters fulfillment and reduces the ego's influence, as our focus turns toward contributing to the greater good.

Relationships offer powerful opportunities for ego transcendence. The ego often seeks to dominate, control, or compete within relationships, leading to conflict and disconnection. By practicing active listening, empathy, and vulnerability, we create space for authentic connection. Recognizing and honoring the perspectives and needs of others reduces the ego's hold, fostering harmony and mutual growth.

Spiritual traditions across cultures emphasize the transcendence of the ego as a path to liberation and enlightenment. In Buddhism, the concept of *anatta* (no-self) teaches that the ego is an illusion, encouraging detachment from identity and desire. In Hinduism, the practice of self-inquiry (*atma vichara*) explores the question "Who am I?" to reveal the true self beyond the ego. These teachings provide timeless guidance for those seeking freedom from the ego's constraints.

Stories of ego transcendence illustrate its transformative power. An individual caught in a cycle of perfectionism finds peace by embracing their imperfections and letting go of the need for approval. A person driven by material success discovers fulfillment in serving others, shifting their focus from accumulation to contribution. A couple experiencing conflict reconnects by releasing blame and practicing mutual understanding, dissolving the ego's need to be "right."

Ultimately, the transcendence of the ego is not about rejecting or defeating it but about integrating it into a larger understanding of the self. The ego becomes a tool rather than a master, supporting our growth and expression without dominating our identity. This integration allows us to live with greater freedom, creativity, and connection.

In transcending the ego, we awaken to the truth of our interconnectedness and the boundless potential within us. We move beyond the limitations of fear and desire, stepping into a life of authenticity, purpose, and unity. This journey is not about becoming something new but remembering and embodying who we truly are—free, whole, and infinite.

Chapter 36
Energetic Connection

The concept of energetic connection reminds us that we are not isolated beings but part of an intricate web of energy that binds all things. This connection extends beyond physical interactions, encompassing the subtle vibrations that flow between individuals, environments, and the universe itself. By understanding and nurturing this connection, we gain insight into how energy shapes our relationships, emotions, and overall well-being, empowering us to live in greater harmony with ourselves and the world around us.

Energetic connection begins with awareness. Everything in existence vibrates at its own unique frequency, from the cells in our bodies to the thoughts in our minds and the spaces we inhabit. These vibrations interact constantly, creating a dynamic exchange of energy. When we become attuned to this flow, we can sense its effects, whether it feels uplifting, draining, or neutral. This awareness allows us to engage with energy more intentionally.

One of the most profound energetic connections is with other people. Humans exchange energy not only through words and actions but also through emotions, body language, and even silence. This exchange can be empowering and inspiring or, in some cases, overwhelming or depleting. Recognizing these energetic dynamics helps us navigate relationships with greater clarity and balance.

Energy cords are a subtle yet powerful aspect of connection. These invisible threads link us to the people, places, and situations we engage with. While some cords are positive, fostering support and love, others can become draining, especially if they are tied to unresolved emotions or unhealthy attachments. Practices like visualization and energy cutting help release cords that no longer serve us, restoring our vitality and focus.

The heart is a central hub of energetic connection. Research shows that the electromagnetic field of the heart is significantly stronger than that of the brain, extending several feet beyond the body. This field plays a vital role in interpersonal connection, influencing how we feel and resonate with others. Practices like heart-focused meditation or expressing gratitude amplify the heart's energy, fostering deeper connections and emotional alignment.

Nature provides a profound source of energetic connection. Walking barefoot on the earth, breathing fresh air, or listening to the sounds of a forest aligns us with the rhythms of the planet, grounding our energy and renewing our vitality. This connection, often referred to as grounding or earthing, reduces stress, calms the mind, and strengthens our bond with the natural world.

Energetic protection is essential for maintaining balance in a connected world. While openness to energy is vital for connection, it's equally important to shield oneself from negative or excessive energies. Techniques such as visualization—imagining a protective light surrounding the body—or carrying grounding tools like crystals can help create energetic boundaries. These practices ensure that we remain centered and resilient in the face of external influences.

Cleansing and renewing our energetic field is another crucial practice. Energy can accumulate in the body and environment, leading to feelings of heaviness or stagnation. Regular cleansing rituals, such as smudging with sage, taking salt baths, or using sound vibrations from singing bowls, clear away stagnant energy and restore balance. These rituals create a fresh, vibrant space for new energy to flow.

Our energetic connection to the spaces we inhabit also profoundly impacts our well-being. Cluttered or chaotic environments can disrupt energy flow, while organized, harmonious spaces promote peace and clarity. Feng Shui and other spatial energy practices provide tools for optimizing the energy of our surroundings, aligning them with our intentions and values.

Intention is a powerful force in energetic connection. By setting clear intentions, we direct our energy purposefully, shaping our interactions and experiences. For example, before entering a conversation, setting an intention to listen with empathy or speak with clarity aligns our energy with these goals. This intentionality fosters meaningful connections and reduces misunderstandings.

Emotions play a key role in energetic connection. High-vibration emotions such as love, joy, and gratitude elevate our energy, attracting positive experiences and relationships. Conversely, lower-vibration emotions like fear or anger can create energetic blockages. While it's natural to experience a range of emotions, practices like mindfulness and emotional processing help us release dense energy and return to balance.

Energetic connection is also deeply spiritual. It reflects our link to the universe, the divine, or the infinite consciousness that underlies all existence. Practices such as prayer, meditation, or simply gazing at the stars remind us of this vast interconnectedness, instilling a sense of wonder and purpose. This connection transcends the individual, uniting us with the collective energy of all life.

Children are often highly attuned to energetic connections. Their openness and sensitivity allow them to sense the energy of people, animals, and spaces more acutely than adults. Encouraging children to trust their instincts and teaching them simple grounding practices helps them navigate these connections while maintaining their sense of wonder and balance.

Energy healing modalities such as Reiki, acupuncture, and chakra balancing directly address the flow of energy within the body. These practices remove blockages, align energy centers, and promote harmony on physical, emotional, and spiritual levels. By working with energy intentionally, these methods support healing and transformation, deepening our connection to ourselves and others.

Technology, while often seen as a barrier to connection, can also be used to foster energetic links. Virtual meditations, online communities, and shared intentions across digital platforms create energetic bonds that transcend physical distance. When used mindfully, technology amplifies connection rather than detracting from it.

Balancing energetic giving and receiving is essential for maintaining healthy connections. Overgiving can lead to depletion, while excessive receiving without reciprocation disrupts harmony. Practices such as expressing gratitude, saying no when necessary, and engaging in acts of kindness create a balanced flow of energy, ensuring mutual nourishment in relationships.

Energetic connection extends to animals and other living beings. Pets, for example, form strong energetic bonds with their human companions, offering unconditional love and emotional support. Spending time with animals or observing wildlife fosters empathy and reminds us of the shared energy that unites all life.

Stories of transformation through energetic connection illustrate its profound impact. A person overwhelmed by toxic relationships finds peace and clarity through energetic boundary work. A family strengthens their bond by creating a shared ritual of gratitude, aligning their energy in harmony. An individual struggling with emotional stagnation renews their vitality through grounding practices in nature.

Ultimately, energetic connection is about unity—recognizing that we are all part of a vast, interconnected field of energy. By nurturing this connection, we align with the flow of life, fostering balance, harmony, and meaning.

In embracing our energetic connection, we deepen our understanding of ourselves and others. We move through the world with greater awareness and compassion, honoring the vibrations that link us to all of existence. This practice is not merely about sensing energy but about living in alignment with it, creating a life of resonance, presence, and purpose.

Chapter 37
Synchronicity and Signs

Synchronicity and signs are subtle yet profound ways the universe communicates with us, guiding us along our paths and affirming our connections to something greater. These meaningful coincidences go beyond chance, often arriving at the perfect moment to provide clarity, confirmation, or encouragement. When we become attuned to these occurrences, we unlock a deeper understanding of life's flow and our role within it.

Synchronicity, a term popularized by psychologist Carl Jung, refers to the simultaneous occurrence of events that appear unrelated yet hold significant meaning when experienced together. Unlike random coincidences, synchronicities evoke a sense of purpose and alignment, as if an unseen force is orchestrating the circumstances. These moments often serve as markers, signaling that we are on the right path or offering guidance during moments of doubt or decision.

Signs, on the other hand, are messages from the universe that may come in various forms—symbols, repeating numbers, animals, songs, or even conversations overheard at the right moment. These signs resonate deeply with the receiver, often carrying a personal significance that defies logic or explanation. Recognizing these signs requires openness, awareness, and trust in their meaning.

To attune ourselves to synchronicities and signs, we must cultivate mindfulness and presence. The fast pace of modern life can desensitize us to the subtle cues the universe provides. Practices like meditation, journaling, or simply pausing to reflect create the space needed to notice and interpret these occurrences.

Being present in the moment sharpens our awareness, allowing us to see connections we might otherwise overlook.

Intuition plays a crucial role in identifying synchronicities and signs. While logic may dismiss these experiences as mere chance, intuition recognizes their deeper significance. This inner knowing often feels like a gentle nudge or a sense of resonance, signaling that something meaningful is at play. Strengthening our intuition through practices like visualization, energy work, or dream journaling enhances our ability to recognize and interpret these messages.

Nature is a common medium for synchronicities and signs. A butterfly landing on your shoulder, the sudden appearance of a rainbow, or the sight of an animal behaving unusually often carries symbolic meaning. Different cultures and traditions attribute specific messages to animals and natural phenomena, but personal interpretation is equally important. For example, seeing a fox might symbolize adaptability and resourcefulness, but for someone with a personal connection to foxes, the message may hold a unique nuance.

Repeating numbers, often referred to as angel numbers, are another powerful form of sign. Patterns like 11:11, 222, or 555 frequently catch our attention and carry specific vibrational meanings. For example, 111 often symbolizes new beginnings and alignment with purpose, while 444 may signify stability and support from the universe. Reflecting on what is happening in your life when you notice these numbers helps uncover their relevance.

Dreams, too, are rich with synchronicities and signs. The dream state provides a direct connection to the subconscious and the universal field, offering symbols, scenarios, or even encounters with loved ones or guides that provide insight and guidance. Keeping a dream journal and exploring recurring themes or emotions enhances our ability to decode these messages and apply them to waking life.

Synchronicities often appear during periods of transition or uncertainty. When we face major life decisions, shifts, or challenges, the universe responds by offering guidance through these meaningful events. For example, meeting someone who shares advice aligned with your current dilemma or stumbling upon a book that addresses your specific question may feel like divine timing. These moments are invitations to trust the unfolding process and take inspired action.

The power of intention amplifies synchronicity. When we set a clear intention—whether through visualization, prayer, or journaling—we align our energy with the desired outcome. This alignment creates a magnetic effect, drawing the people, opportunities, and circumstances needed to manifest our goals. Synchronicities then act as markers, confirming that our energy and actions are in alignment with our intentions.

Signs and synchronicities also foster trust in the universe. By observing how events unfold in perfect timing, we strengthen our belief in a higher intelligence at work. This trust reduces the need for control and cultivates a sense of surrender, allowing us to flow with life's rhythms rather than resist them.

Interpreting synchronicities and signs is a deeply personal process. While some symbols hold universal meanings, their significance often depends on the context of the individual's life. For example, a recurring song might remind one person of a lost loved one, while for another, it may represent a call to action. Paying attention to emotions and intuitive impressions provides clarity about the message's meaning.

Rituals and practices can enhance our connection to signs and synchronicities. Creating a gratitude journal for moments of synchronicity acknowledges and amplifies these experiences. Lighting a candle, meditating, or performing a short ceremony when asking for guidance invites clarity and strengthens our relationship with the unseen forces at play.

Sharing stories of synchronicity with others often reveals how common these experiences are. A friend might share how meeting someone on a whim led to an unexpected career opportunity, while another recounts how a random encounter provided the exact advice they needed. These stories remind us that we are part of a larger interconnected web, where even the smallest events carry profound meaning.

Children, with their open minds and unfiltered curiosity, are particularly attuned to synchronicities and signs. Encouraging children to notice and share these moments fosters their intuitive abilities and nurtures a sense of wonder about the world. Observing how children perceive these occurrences can also inspire adults to reconnect with their own sense of trust and openness.

While synchronicities and signs often feel magical, they are not meant to replace personal responsibility or decision-making. Instead, they serve as guides, offering reassurance and insight while empowering us to take aligned action. By combining these messages with our own wisdom and discernment, we co-create our paths with the universe.

Stories of transformation through synchronicities and signs highlight their life-changing impact. A person feeling lost and disconnected begins noticing recurring symbols that lead them to a new passion or purpose. A traveler struggling with doubt meets a stranger who shares wisdom that resolves their uncertainty. An artist battling creative block finds inspiration in an unexpected coincidence that sparks their next masterpiece.

Ultimately, synchronicities and signs remind us that we are not alone in our journey. They affirm that the universe is responsive, offering guidance, support, and connection at every step. By attuning ourselves to these messages, we align with the flow of life, embracing its mystery and magic.

In recognizing and honoring synchronicities and signs, we deepen our connection to the unseen forces that shape our lives. These moments become more than fleeting curiosities; they become sacred markers of alignment, trust, and purpose. Through this awareness, we learn to move through life with open eyes, open hearts, and a profound sense of connection to the greater whole.

Chapter 38
Intuition and Wisdom

Intuition is one of the most profound gifts of the human experience—a quiet, inner knowing that transcends logic and connects us to universal wisdom. Often called the "inner compass" or "gut feeling," intuition is a guiding force that helps us navigate life's complexities with clarity and confidence. Cultivating and trusting intuition enables us to access insights that align us with our true selves and the flow of life.

Intuition is not a mysterious ability reserved for the few; it is an inherent quality within everyone. It arises from the interconnectedness of the mind, body, and spirit, offering guidance that integrates conscious thought with subconscious awareness. Unlike the analytical mind, which seeks linear reasoning and proof, intuition speaks in subtle impressions, feelings, and images. It is a sense that transcends words, often arriving as a certainty that defies explanation.

Developing intuition begins with listening. In a world filled with noise and distraction, the voice of intuition can be drowned out by external influences and internal doubts. Quieting the mind through practices like meditation, breathwork, or time spent in nature creates the space needed to hear this inner guidance. These moments of stillness sharpen our ability to sense and trust the intuitive nudges that arise.

The body is a powerful ally in accessing intuition. Physical sensations often accompany intuitive messages—such as a sense of warmth in the chest, a tingle in the spine, or a sudden sense of calm. Learning to recognize and interpret these sensations strengthens the connection between intuition and decision-making. For instance, a feeling of tension might signal misalignment, while ease or excitement may indicate the right path.

Dreams are another gateway to intuition. The dream state allows the subconscious mind to communicate through symbols, scenarios, and emotions. Keeping a dream journal and reflecting on recurring themes or vivid imagery offers valuable insights into unresolved questions or emerging possibilities. Dreams often provide answers that the waking mind struggles to uncover.

Trust is essential in working with intuition. Many people dismiss their intuitive feelings, fearing they may be wrong or irrational. Yet, intuition often speaks before logic can process a situation, offering truths that only become clear in hindsight. Building trust in this inner knowing involves taking small steps—acting on intuitive guidance in minor decisions and observing the outcomes. Over time, these experiences affirm the reliability of intuition, building confidence in its wisdom.

Creativity is deeply linked to intuition. Artists, writers, and innovators often describe their creative process as intuitive—a flow state where ideas and solutions seem to arise effortlessly. Engaging in creative activities without judgment or expectation allows intuition to emerge naturally. Whether painting, writing, or brainstorming, these moments of openness invite intuitive insights to guide the process.

Journaling is a practical tool for strengthening intuition. Writing down thoughts, feelings, and questions creates a dialogue with the inner self, allowing intuitive responses to surface. Stream-of-consciousness writing, where words flow without overthinking, often reveals surprising insights and connections. Reviewing past entries can also highlight patterns or recurring themes, providing clarity about intuitive guidance.

Nature enhances intuitive awareness by reconnecting us to the rhythms and cycles of the earth. Walking in a forest, observing the ocean's waves, or simply sitting under a tree fosters a sense of harmony and openness. These moments of connection quiet the analytical mind and awaken the intuitive, allowing us to feel more attuned to the flow of life.

Intuition is closely tied to the heart. While the mind seeks logic, the heart senses truth. Practices that focus on the heart—such as gratitude meditation, heart-centered breathing, or simply placing a hand over the chest while reflecting—strengthen this connection. The heart often provides answers that feel deeply aligned, even if they challenge conventional reasoning.

Intuition also plays a critical role in relationships. It allows us to sense unspoken emotions, discern intentions, and navigate complex dynamics. For instance, intuition might alert us to a hidden tension in a conversation or guide us toward deeper understanding and empathy. Trusting these feelings fosters stronger, more authentic connections.

Energy practices such as Reiki, chakra balancing, or breathwork clear energetic blockages that can hinder intuitive flow. When energy flows freely, we become more receptive to the subtle cues of intuition. These practices also raise our vibrational frequency, aligning us with the universal energy that fuels intuitive insight.

For those seeking guidance on major life decisions, intuition provides a powerful compass. By tuning into how different choices feel—rather than solely analyzing their pros and cons—we access a deeper wisdom. Visualization exercises, where we imagine ourselves living each potential outcome, often reveal which path resonates most deeply with our inner truth.

Children naturally embody intuitive wisdom. They act on instinct, express feelings without overanalyzing, and often notice details adults overlook. Encouraging children to trust their feelings, ask questions, and explore their curiosities nurtures their intuitive abilities. Adults can learn from this innate openness, reclaiming their own intuitive instincts through observation and practice.

Balancing intuition with logic creates a harmonious decision-making process. While intuition provides insight, logic helps ground those insights in practical action. For example, an intuitive nudge to pursue a new career might be followed by research and planning. This integration ensures that intuitive guidance is both honored and effectively implemented.

Stories of intuition transforming lives demonstrate its profound impact. A person uncertain about a career path feels an intuitive pull toward a creative pursuit, leading to unexpected success. A traveler senses they should delay a trip, avoiding unforeseen challenges. A parent instinctively knows how to comfort their child in a moment of distress. These examples show how intuition guides us toward alignment and connection.

Ultimately, intuition is a bridge to universal wisdom. It transcends the limitations of the rational mind, connecting us to a vast field of knowledge that is always available. By cultivating this connection, we align with the flow of life, making decisions with clarity and confidence.

In embracing intuition, we honor the wisdom within and around us. We move through life with greater trust, authenticity, and presence, guided by a force that transcends explanation yet feels undeniably true. This journey deepens our connection to ourselves, others, and the infinite intelligence of the universe, reminding us that we are never truly lost—only learning to listen more closely.

Chapter 39
Holism and Modernity

The modern world is defined by speed, complexity, and an ever-increasing reliance on technology. While these advancements bring convenience and progress, they often create a disconnection from the natural rhythms of life and the deeper aspects of our existence. Holism, with its emphasis on balance, interconnectedness, and mindful living, offers a transformative lens through which to navigate the challenges and opportunities of modernity.

Holism in modernity begins with redefining success. In a world that often equates achievement with productivity and material gain, the holistic approach emphasizes well-being, purpose, and alignment. Success is no longer measured solely by external accomplishments but by the harmony between personal growth, relationships, and contribution to the greater good. This shift encourages individuals to prioritize what truly matters, fostering a sense of fulfillment beyond superficial metrics.

Technology, one of the most influential forces of modern life, is a double-edged sword. It connects people across the globe, provides access to infinite knowledge, and facilitates innovation, but it also fosters distractions, shallow connections, and information overload. Holism invites a mindful relationship with technology, encouraging its use as a tool for growth, connection, and creativity rather than an unconscious habit or escape. Setting boundaries—such as designated screen-free times or intentional digital detoxes—helps reclaim focus and presence.

The rise of urban living presents another modern challenge to holistic living. Cities, with their density and fast-paced environments, can feel disconnected from nature and inner peace. Integrating green spaces into urban settings, practicing mindfulness amidst noise, and seeking moments of stillness in the chaos help restore balance. Even small acts, like growing plants on a balcony or walking in a park, reconnect urban dwellers to the natural world.

Work-life balance is a significant concern in modernity, as careers often demand long hours and constant availability. The holistic perspective emphasizes the importance of aligning work with values and creating space for rest, relationships, and personal interests. This balance is not about achieving perfection but about honoring the ebb and flow of energy, recognizing when to push forward and when to recharge. Flexible schedules, mindfulness practices, and prioritizing mental health are key strategies for achieving this harmony.

Holistic health in the modern era addresses the interplay between physical, mental, and emotional well-being. Fast food, sedentary lifestyles, and stress are pervasive challenges, but a holistic approach counters these with mindful eating, movement, and stress management techniques. Practices like yoga, meditation, and energy healing integrate ancient wisdom with modern needs, offering tools for resilience and vitality.

Education in the modern world is often focused on academic achievement and technical skills, sometimes at the expense of emotional and spiritual growth. Holistic education promotes a balanced approach, nurturing creativity, empathy, and critical thinking alongside intellectual development. Programs that incorporate mindfulness, outdoor learning, and emotional intelligence cultivate well-rounded individuals equipped to thrive in a complex world.

The digital age has transformed communication, enabling instantaneous connections but often reducing the depth of relationships. Holistic communication emphasizes authenticity, active listening, and empathy, creating meaningful interactions even in virtual spaces. Simple practices, like mindful conversations or expressing gratitude, strengthen bonds and counteract the superficiality of modern communication norms.

Sustainability is a pressing issue in modernity, as rapid industrialization and consumerism strain the planet's resources. Holism aligns closely with sustainable living, advocating for conscious consumption, renewable energy, and ecological stewardship. Practices like minimalism, zero-waste living, and supporting ethical businesses reflect a commitment to the interconnected well-being of humans and the environment.

Modernity also brings opportunities for holistic growth. The accessibility of knowledge through books, podcasts, and online courses allows individuals to explore diverse perspectives and deepen their understanding of holistic principles. Communities—both local and global—centered on mindfulness, wellness, and sustainability provide support and inspiration for those seeking to integrate holism into their lives.

Social media, often criticized for its negative impact, can be a tool for spreading holistic values when used intentionally. Platforms that share content on mindfulness, health, and environmental advocacy inspire positive change. Following accounts aligned with one's values and limiting exposure to negative or superficial content creates a more uplifting digital environment.

The modern fast-paced lifestyle often leads to stress and burnout, making rest and relaxation essential. Holism views rest not as a luxury but as a necessity for balance and renewal. Practices like restorative yoga, nature retreats, and mindful sleep rituals help counteract the effects of chronic stress, restoring vitality and clarity.

Spirituality in modernity often takes on a more individualized and inclusive form. While traditional religions continue to provide guidance for many, holistic spirituality focuses on personal exploration, interconnectedness, and universal values. Practices like meditation, breathwork, and energy healing transcend cultural and religious boundaries, offering accessible paths to inner peace and connection.

Children in the modern world face unique challenges, from screen addiction to overstimulation. Raising children holistically involves fostering their natural curiosity, creativity, and emotional intelligence. Encouraging outdoor play, teaching mindfulness, and modeling balanced digital use provide children with tools to navigate modernity with resilience and joy.

Holistic leadership is increasingly relevant in the modern workplace. Leaders who prioritize empathy, collaboration, and sustainability inspire teams to align with shared values and purpose. This approach transforms organizations from profit-driven entities into communities that value well-being, innovation, and positive impact.

Nature remains a grounding force amidst the complexities of modern life. Practices like forest bathing, gardening, or simply observing the changing seasons restore perspective and calm. These moments of connection remind us that, despite technological advances, we are still deeply tied to the natural rhythms of the earth.

The challenges of modernity often highlight the need for simplicity. Holism encourages a return to essentials, focusing on what truly nourishes the soul. This might involve decluttering physical spaces, simplifying schedules, or embracing slow living. By letting go of excess, we create room for meaning and joy.

Stories of individuals integrating holism into modern life illustrate its transformative potential. A corporate executive finds balance by practicing meditation and prioritizing time with family. A city dweller reconnects with nature through weekend hikes and a rooftop garden. A student balances academic pressure with daily mindfulness practices, enhancing focus and well-being.

Ultimately, holism in modernity is about conscious integration. It does not reject progress or technology but seeks to align them with values of balance, connection, and sustainability. By approaching modern challenges with a holistic mindset, we create a life that honors both our individual needs and the collective good.

In embracing holism, we transform modernity from a source of stress and disconnection into an opportunity for growth and alignment. By living with intention and awareness, we bridge the gap between the ancient and the contemporary, creating a world that is not only efficient but also meaningful, connected, and whole.

Chapter 40
Nocturnal Practices

The hours of the night hold a unique energy—quiet, introspective, and restorative. They offer a time to slow down, reflect, and reconnect with our inner selves. Nocturnal practices, designed to align with this tranquil energy, can transform the night into a sacred space for healing, growth, and renewal. These rituals not only prepare the body and mind for restful sleep but also open the doorway to deeper awareness and insight through dreams and stillness.

One of the simplest yet most powerful nocturnal practices is creating a calming evening routine. The hours leading up to bedtime set the tone for the quality of rest and the state of the subconscious mind. A consistent routine signals the body to transition from the busyness of the day into relaxation. Activities such as dimming lights, disconnecting from screens, or engaging in light stretching prepare the nervous system for sleep, fostering a sense of peace.

Breathwork is an essential tool for unwinding at night. Simple breathing exercises, like inhaling for a count of four, holding for four, and exhaling for four, calm the mind and body. This practice reduces stress hormones, slows the heart rate, and encourages a state of relaxation. Incorporating breath awareness into an evening ritual anchors the mind in the present moment, easing the transition to rest.

Meditation before sleep allows the mind to release the worries and thoughts accumulated during the day. Guided meditations focused on relaxation, body scans, or visualization are particularly effective for quieting the inner chatter. A brief practice of gratitude meditation—reflecting on the day's blessings and lessons—cultivates positive emotions, creating a peaceful mental state for sleep.

Journaling is another practice that promotes mental clarity at night. Writing down thoughts, emotions, or reflections provides a space to process the day's events, clearing the mind before sleep. A "worry journal" can be particularly helpful for those who struggle with racing thoughts at night—simply jotting down concerns and affirming that they will be addressed the next day allows the mind to let go and relax.

Rituals involving the senses help create a soothing nighttime environment. Aromatherapy, using essential oils like lavender, chamomile, or sandalwood, calms the nervous system and prepares the mind for rest. Soft lighting, such as candles or salt lamps, creates a gentle ambiance. Listening to calming music, nature sounds, or binaural beats aligns the mind with slower, more restful brainwave frequencies, promoting deep relaxation.

Dreamwork is a profound aspect of nocturnal practices. The dream state offers access to the subconscious mind, providing insight, creativity, and healing. Setting an intention before sleep—such as seeking clarity on a question or asking for guidance—often influences the themes and messages of dreams. Keeping a dream journal by the bedside encourages immediate recording of dreams upon waking, preserving their details and facilitating deeper reflection.

For those interested in lucid dreaming—the ability to become aware and even influence the dream state—nocturnal practices take on an additional layer of purpose. Techniques such as reality checks during the day (questioning whether one is awake or dreaming) or affirming intentions for lucidity before sleep heighten the likelihood of conscious dreaming. Lucid dreaming opens doors to exploration, creativity, and self-discovery within the dream world.

Body care rituals promote relaxation and physical comfort before sleep. Warm baths with Epsom salts or calming herbs like lavender relax tense muscles and draw out stress. Self-massage with soothing oils nourishes the skin and provides a grounding, nurturing experience. These practices align the body with the night's restorative energy, preparing it for deep rest.

Sleep hygiene is a cornerstone of nocturnal well-being. Ensuring that the sleep environment is cool, quiet, and free of distractions creates the optimal conditions for rest. Investing in a comfortable mattress and natural bedding materials supports physical relaxation. Blackout curtains or sleep masks block out light, while white noise machines or earplugs reduce disruptions from sound.

The relationship between the moon and nocturnal practices is significant. The moon's phases influence energy levels and emotions, offering opportunities to align practices with its cycles. The new moon encourages introspection and intention-setting, while the full moon amplifies reflection, gratitude, and release. Spending time under moonlight or incorporating moon rituals into nighttime routines deepens the connection to this celestial rhythm.

For those who experience insomnia or disrupted sleep, holistic approaches provide gentle remedies. Herbal teas made with chamomile, valerian root, or passionflower calm the mind and body. Acupressure or yoga poses like child's pose or legs-up-the-wall release physical tension and encourage relaxation. Exploring the underlying emotional or energetic causes of sleeplessness through journaling or therapy brings awareness and healing to these patterns.

Nocturnal practices are also an opportunity to deepen spiritual connection. Prayer, contemplation, or connecting with guides or ancestors through quiet reflection fosters a sense of presence and support. These practices transform the night into a sacred time for aligning with the divine, fostering inner peace and trust.

The power of intention shapes the energy of the night. Before sleep, affirming a positive focus—such as "I release what no longer serves me" or "I welcome rest and renewal"—sets the tone for the subconscious mind. These intentions act as seeds, influencing both the dream state and the emotional energy carried into the next day.

Children benefit greatly from gentle nocturnal practices. Reading bedtime stories, practicing gratitude, or engaging in light stretching help children wind down and establish healthy sleep habits. Incorporating sensory elements like soft lighting or calming music creates a nurturing environment that supports their emotional and physical well-being.

For couples, nocturnal practices can strengthen intimacy and connection. Sharing gratitude for one another, engaging in synchronized breathing exercises, or holding hands during meditation fosters emotional closeness. These rituals create a space for deepening the bond while honoring the restorative energy of the night.

Stories of transformation through nocturnal practices reveal their profound impact. A busy professional discovers that a nightly gratitude journal reduces stress and improves sleep. A parent finds solace in moonlit meditation, balancing the demands of the day with moments of peace. An artist reignites their creativity by engaging in dreamwork, uncovering inspiration through symbolic messages.

Ultimately, nocturnal practices are about honoring the natural rhythms of rest and renewal. They transform the night from a time of mere inactivity into a sacred space for healing, reflection, and connection. By embracing these practices, we align with the wisdom of the night, creating a foundation for well-being that carries into the day.

In reclaiming the night as a time of restoration and insight, we cultivate a deeper relationship with ourselves and the universe. These practices remind us that even in stillness, growth and transformation occur, inviting us to embrace the beauty and power of the dark hours as part of life's holistic journey.

Chapter 41
Transgenerational Healing

Transgenerational healing addresses the patterns, emotions, and energy that are passed down through generations, shaping the lives of descendants in ways that often go unnoticed. These inherited dynamics can include unresolved traumas, limiting beliefs, or emotional imbalances that influence how individuals think, feel, and act. By identifying and transforming these inherited patterns, transgenerational healing offers an opportunity for profound liberation—not only for the individual but for their lineage and future generations.

At its core, transgenerational healing begins with awareness. Each family carries its unique energetic imprint, shaped by the experiences, choices, and traumas of its members. These imprints often manifest in recurring themes—such as struggles with relationships, financial instability, or emotional repression—that are repeated across generations. Becoming aware of these patterns is the first step in breaking free from their influence.

One of the most common ways generational patterns are transmitted is through emotional energy. Traumas experienced by ancestors, such as loss, war, or displacement, leave energetic imprints that can be passed down through both stories and silence. For instance, a family with a history of suppressed grief may unknowingly perpetuate an emotional avoidance pattern. Recognizing these dynamics allows individuals to begin the process of healing and releasing.

Family stories and cultural narratives often provide clues about transgenerational patterns. Reflecting on shared family experiences—such as beliefs about money, expressions of love, or approaches to conflict—can reveal underlying themes. For example, a family that repeatedly tells stories of scarcity may unknowingly reinforce limiting beliefs about abundance. By identifying these narratives, individuals can rewrite them with empowering perspectives.

Ancestral trauma can also be inherited biologically. Studies in epigenetics suggest that the experiences of our ancestors can influence gene expression, affecting how we respond to stress or regulate emotions. This scientific insight reinforces the importance of addressing inherited patterns holistically, combining emotional, energetic, and biological approaches to healing.

One powerful tool for transgenerational healing is the practice of family constellations. This therapeutic approach explores the hidden dynamics within a family system, uncovering unresolved emotions or imbalances that are affecting descendants. Through guided visualization and symbolic representation, participants gain insight into these dynamics and work toward resolution, often experiencing a sense of release and clarity.

Forgiveness plays a central role in transgenerational healing. This includes forgiving ancestors for the pain they may have caused—whether consciously or unconsciously—and forgiving oneself for perpetuating patterns. Forgiveness is not about condoning harm but about releasing the energetic weight of resentment, allowing for greater freedom and compassion.

Rituals and ceremonies offer another avenue for ancestral healing. Lighting candles, offering prayers, or creating altars in honor of ancestors create spaces for connection and healing. These acts acknowledge the struggles and strengths of those who came before us, fostering a sense of gratitude and closure. For instance, a ritual of releasing—such as writing down an inherited belief and symbolically burning it—can mark the end of a limiting cycle.

Dreamwork can also reveal transgenerational influences. Ancestors often appear in dreams as guides or messengers, offering insights into unresolved family dynamics. Keeping a dream journal and reflecting on the emotions or symbols that arise helps uncover the deeper meanings of these nocturnal encounters, guiding the healing process.

Energy healing modalities such as Reiki, chakra balancing, or shamanic practices address the energetic imprints of ancestral trauma. By working with the body's energy field, these practices clear blockages and restore balance, allowing individuals to release inherited patterns. Techniques like soul retrieval or cord-cutting ceremonies can further sever ties to unhealthy ancestral energies, promoting renewal and empowerment.

Engaging in creative expression—through art, music, or writing—provides a channel for processing and transforming inherited emotions. For instance, painting a family tree with symbols representing both strengths and challenges can create a visual representation of healing. Poetry or journaling allows individuals to give voice to emotions that may have been suppressed across generations, fostering understanding and release.

Community and support are vital in transgenerational healing. Sharing stories and experiences within a group or with a trusted therapist creates a sense of solidarity and validation. Knowing that others are also navigating inherited patterns fosters courage and resilience, reminding individuals that they are not alone in this journey.

Nature serves as a grounding force during the healing process. Spending time in natural environments, such as forests or by water, provides a sense of renewal and connection to the broader cycles of life. Practices like walking meditations or tree-honoring rituals symbolize the strength and rootedness of family lineage while encouraging the release of burdens.

Children benefit profoundly from transgenerational healing. By addressing inherited patterns, parents and caregivers create a healthier emotional environment for future generations. Teaching children about the strengths and resilience of their ancestors, while also encouraging emotional expression and individuality, helps them build a balanced sense of identity.

The benefits of transgenerational healing extend beyond the individual. As one person heals, they create ripples of change within the family system, influencing relationships and dynamics in positive ways. This process not only honors the struggles of ancestors but also empowers future generations to live with greater freedom, balance, and joy.

Stories of transformation through transgenerational healing illustrate its profound impact. A woman burdened by perfectionism discovers its roots in her grandmother's need for control during times of chaos, allowing her to release the pattern and embrace self-compassion. A man estranged from his father reconciles after uncovering the shared pain passed down through their lineage. A family breaks free from cycles of poverty by rewriting inherited beliefs about abundance and worthiness.

Ultimately, transgenerational healing is about reclaiming agency over our lives. It honors the struggles and strengths of those who came before us while freeing us to create our own paths. This process is not about erasing the past but about transforming its energy into a source of wisdom and empowerment.

In healing the wounds of the past, we not only liberate ourselves but also contribute to the healing of our families and communities. Transgenerational healing reminds us that we are both shaped by our lineage and capable of shaping it, creating a legacy of resilience, love, and possibility for the generations to come.

Chapter 42
Collective Energy

Collective energy refers to the shared vibrational field created by the emotions, intentions, and actions of individuals within a group, community, or even the entire world. It is an invisible yet powerful force that can influence societal dynamics, individual well-being, and global outcomes. By understanding and consciously contributing to collective energy, we can harness its potential to create positive change, foster unity, and elevate humanity as a whole.

The concept of collective energy is rooted in the idea that we are all interconnected. Just as individual energy influences those in our immediate environment, collective energy operates on a larger scale, impacting communities, nations, and the planet. This shared field is shaped by the thoughts, emotions, and actions of each person, creating a feedback loop that amplifies both positive and negative energies.

Awareness of collective energy begins with recognizing its presence in everyday life. Consider the atmosphere of a crowded concert, where excitement and joy are palpable, or the tension in a room following a disagreement. These experiences reflect the power of collective energy to influence mood, behavior, and connection. On a global scale, events like natural disasters or celebrations of unity evoke shared emotional responses, reinforcing the bonds between individuals.

One of the most significant ways we contribute to collective energy is through our emotional state. Emotions such as love, gratitude, and compassion elevate the vibrational frequency of the collective field, fostering harmony and resilience.

Conversely, fear, anger, and despair can create waves of negativity that spread beyond the individual. By cultivating awareness of our emotional energy and intentionally raising our vibration, we become agents of positive change within the collective.

Meditation and mindfulness practices play a vital role in shaping collective energy. Group meditations, whether in person or virtual, amplify the energy of peace, healing, and unity, creating ripples that extend far beyond the participants. Studies have shown that large-scale meditations can reduce crime rates and promote social harmony in surrounding areas, highlighting the tangible impact of collective intention.

Shared intentions are another powerful way to influence collective energy. When groups align their focus on a specific goal—such as healing, peace, or environmental sustainability—they create a unified energetic force that strengthens the likelihood of achieving that goal. Ceremonies, prayers, or synchronized actions amplify this effect, reinforcing the collective field with clarity and purpose.

The energy of gratitude is particularly transformative within the collective. Expressing appreciation for others, nature, or shared experiences generates a ripple effect, inspiring more acts of kindness and connection. Gratitude circles, where individuals share what they are thankful for, elevate the emotional tone of groups, fostering a sense of belonging and mutual support.

Collective energy is also deeply tied to the natural world. The earth itself has an energetic frequency, often referred to as the Schumann resonance, which is influenced by human activity and emotions. Practices like tree-planting initiatives, environmental cleanups, or rituals honoring the earth not only restore ecosystems but also harmonize collective energy with the planet's rhythms.

Technology has become a conduit for collective energy in the modern world. Social media, virtual gatherings, and online campaigns connect individuals across the globe, creating opportunities for shared intention and action. However, technology also amplifies negativity when used without mindfulness, spreading fear or division. By consciously curating our digital interactions and focusing on uplifting content, we contribute to a more positive collective energy online.

Crises and challenges often reveal the strength of collective energy. During times of hardship, communities come together to support one another, generating waves of compassion and resilience. These moments demonstrate humanity's capacity to unite, reminding us of the profound power of shared purpose and connection.

Balancing the collective energy of a group requires addressing both positive and negative dynamics. For instance, in workplaces or communities where tension or conflict arises, practices like open dialogue, active listening, and mutual respect help realign the group's energy. Leaders play a crucial role in setting the energetic tone, modeling behaviors that promote inclusion, collaboration, and empathy.

Healing collective wounds is an essential aspect of elevating collective energy. Historical injustices, cultural traumas, and systemic imbalances create energetic imprints that perpetuate division and pain. Acknowledging and addressing these wounds—through education, reconciliation, and restorative practices—creates opportunities for healing and transformation. By honoring the past while committing to a more equitable future, we shift the collective energy toward unity and growth.

Children are especially sensitive to collective energy. They often absorb the emotional tone of their surroundings, whether at home, school, or in society. Creating supportive, loving environments for children nurtures their well-being and ensures they contribute positively to the collective field as they grow. Teaching children mindfulness, kindness, and empathy equips them to navigate and influence collective energy with awareness.

Art and creativity are powerful mediums for elevating collective energy. Music, visual art, and storytelling have the ability to transcend differences, evoking shared emotions and inspiring collective reflection. Festivals, performances, and collaborative projects bring people together, fostering joy, connection, and understanding.

The relationship between individual and collective energy is reciprocal. While collective energy influences the individual, each person's energy also contributes to the whole. This interconnectedness underscores the importance of personal responsibility in shaping the collective field. By cultivating inner balance, authenticity, and compassion, we ripple these qualities outward, uplifting those around us.

Stories of collective energy transforming communities highlight its potential. A city ravaged by disaster rebuilds stronger than before through shared resilience and mutual support. A global meditation event inspires millions to focus on peace, creating measurable decreases in violence. A grassroots movement for environmental conservation sparks worldwide awareness and action, proving that collective intention can lead to profound change.

Ultimately, collective energy reminds us of our shared humanity and interconnectedness. It is a force that transcends borders, beliefs, and differences, uniting us in the pursuit of a better world. By consciously contributing to the collective field, we become co-creators of a future rooted in love, harmony, and purpose.

In aligning with positive collective energy, we honor our role as stewards of the world we share. This practice invites us to act with intention, empathy, and courage, knowing that our individual energy is a vital thread in the vast, interconnected tapestry of life. Together, we have the power to shape a collective energy that uplifts, heals, and inspires generations to come.

Chapter 43
The Hero's Journey

The hero's journey is a timeless metaphor for personal transformation and the holistic path to self-discovery. Rooted in mythology and storytelling, it describes the arc of a protagonist who faces challenges, overcomes obstacles, and emerges transformed. In the context of holistic living, the hero's journey represents the process of awakening to our true potential, embracing growth, and integrating lessons into a life of purpose and alignment.

Every hero's journey begins with a call to adventure. This call often arises as a sense of dissatisfaction with the status quo—a longing for deeper meaning, a desire for change, or a challenge that disrupts the familiar. In the holistic journey, this might take the form of a health crisis, a spiritual awakening, or a moment of profound introspection. The call is an invitation to step into the unknown and explore the deeper aspects of the self.

The initial response to the call is often resistance. The hero may feel fear, doubt, or a reluctance to leave the comfort of the familiar. In holistic living, this resistance might manifest as clinging to old habits, limiting beliefs, or fear of the unknown. Yet, within this resistance lies an opportunity for growth. By recognizing these fears as natural and necessary, we build the courage to take the first step forward.

The journey truly begins when the hero crosses the threshold from the known into the unknown. This transition marks a departure from the familiar and an embrace of the mysteries ahead. In holistic terms, crossing the threshold might involve committing to a new practice, exploring uncharted aspects of spirituality, or embarking on a healing journey. This step requires trust in oneself and the process, even in the face of uncertainty.

As the hero ventures deeper into the journey, they encounter allies and mentors who provide guidance, support, and wisdom. These figures often appear as teachers, friends, or spiritual guides, offering tools and insights that help the hero navigate challenges. In holistic living, mentors might take the form of yoga instructors, therapists, or even books and experiences that resonate deeply. The presence of allies reminds us that we are not alone in our journey.

Challenges and trials are an integral part of the hero's journey. These obstacles test the hero's resolve, forcing them to confront their fears, doubts, and inner shadows. In holistic living, these trials might include moments of self-doubt, emotional upheaval, or setbacks in progress. Yet, each challenge serves as a teacher, offering lessons and strengthening the hero's resilience. Facing these trials with courage and authenticity leads to profound growth.

The hero often encounters a pivotal moment of transformation, referred to as the "abyss" or "dark night of the soul." This is a time of intense inner struggle, where old identities, beliefs, or patterns are confronted and released. In holistic terms, this might involve a deep healing process, a spiritual awakening, or a moment of surrender. While this phase is often the most difficult, it is also the most transformative, marking the beginning of a new chapter in the hero's journey.

Emerging from the abyss, the hero experiences a rebirth—a renewed sense of self and purpose. This stage represents the integration of lessons learned and the discovery of inner strength and wisdom. In holistic living, rebirth might manifest as a sense of clarity, alignment, or peace. The hero realizes that the journey was not about external achievements but about the transformation of the inner world.

The return home is the final stage of the hero's journey. The hero brings back the wisdom, insights, and growth gained during their adventure, sharing these gifts with their community. In holistic living, this might involve mentoring others, contributing to collective healing, or simply living authentically. The return is not a return to the same life, but a return to life transformed—infused with the awareness gained through the journey.

The hero's journey is not a linear path but a cyclical one. Each stage prepares the hero for the next adventure, as growth and transformation are ongoing processes. In holistic living, this cycle reflects the natural rhythms of life—periods of expansion, contraction, and renewal. Embracing this flow allows us to approach challenges and transitions with grace and trust.

Symbols play a significant role in the hero's journey. Objects, places, or experiences often carry deep meaning, serving as reminders of the hero's purpose and transformation. In holistic practices, symbols like mandalas, crystals, or sacred spaces hold similar significance, anchoring us in the present moment and connecting us to the greater journey of life.

Stories of the hero's journey inspire us to see our own lives as epic narratives of growth and transformation. Consider the individual who overcomes a health crisis to inspire others with their resilience or the person who embarks on a spiritual quest and returns with a renewed sense of purpose. These stories remind us that challenges are not roadblocks but stepping stones on the path to self-discovery.

Children naturally embody the spirit of the hero's journey. Their curiosity, courage, and openness to learning mirror the qualities of a hero embarking on an adventure. Encouraging children to explore, ask questions, and embrace challenges nurtures their inner hero and prepares them for the cycles of growth they will encounter throughout life.

The hero's journey is also reflected in the collective experience. Movements for social justice, environmental sustainability, or global healing often mirror this arc, with communities answering a call to action, facing challenges, and emerging transformed. These collective journeys demonstrate the power of shared purpose and remind us of the interconnectedness of all life.

Ultimately, the hero's journey is about awakening to our fullest potential. It invites us to step beyond fear and limitation, embracing the unknown with curiosity and trust. Along the way, we discover not only who we are but also the infinite possibilities that lie within us.

In recognizing our own lives as hero's journeys, we honor the challenges, triumphs, and transformations that shape us. We see each moment—whether joyful or difficult—as part of a larger narrative of growth and connection. By embracing this perspective, we step into our roles as the heroes of our own stories, co-creating a life of meaning, purpose, and authenticity.

Chapter 44
Expansion of Consciousness

The expansion of consciousness is a profound journey of awakening, a process of broadening one's awareness beyond the immediate and tangible to perceive the interconnectedness of all things. It is a shift from living solely in the physical, logical realm to embracing a deeper understanding of spiritual truths, universal energy, and the boundless potential of the human mind. This journey is not a destination but a continuous unfolding, a limitless process of growth and discovery.

At its core, consciousness is the essence of our awareness—our ability to perceive, experience, and respond to life. In its expanded state, consciousness transcends the confines of the ego and the linear mind, allowing us to access higher states of being and a greater sense of connection to the universe. This expansion enhances our capacity for empathy, creativity, intuition, and spiritual insight.

The process of expanding consciousness often begins with a shift in perspective. A moment of awe in nature, a profound meditation, or an experience of synchronicity can serve as a catalyst, breaking through the layers of routine perception and inviting us to explore deeper truths. These moments act as doorways, revealing glimpses of the vast, interconnected reality that lies beyond everyday awareness.

Meditation is one of the most effective tools for expanding consciousness. By quieting the mind and focusing inward, we create space for higher awareness to emerge. Techniques such as mindfulness, transcendental meditation, or chakra-focused practices open the mind and heart, enabling us to access states of inner peace and universal connection. Over time, these practices shift our baseline consciousness, allowing us to live with greater clarity and presence.

Breathwork is another powerful practice for expanding consciousness. Conscious breathing techniques, such as deep diaphragmatic breathing or holotropic breathwork, alter our state of awareness by activating the body's energy centers and calming the nervous system. These practices often lead to transformative insights, emotional releases, and heightened spiritual awareness.

Dream states also play a role in expanding consciousness. During sleep, the conscious mind relaxes, allowing the subconscious to communicate through symbols, scenarios, and emotions. Lucid dreaming—where one becomes aware of the dream state and can actively participate—provides an opportunity to explore consciousness beyond the waking mind. Journaling dreams and reflecting on their meanings deepen this exploration.

Psychedelic experiences, when approached responsibly and in the right context, have been used for millennia to facilitate expanded states of consciousness. Indigenous cultures have long utilized plant medicines like ayahuasca, peyote, or psilocybin for spiritual growth and healing. These substances can dissolve the boundaries of the ego, offering profound insights into the nature of existence. However, these experiences should always be undertaken with proper guidance, preparation, and respect for their power.

Nature serves as a gateway to expanded consciousness. The rhythms of the earth, the vastness of the sky, and the intricate beauty of ecosystems remind us of the unity and intelligence inherent in all life. Practices like forest bathing, stargazing, or simply sitting in silence amidst natural surroundings align us with the flow of the universe, grounding us while simultaneously opening us to greater awareness.

Sacred geometry and symbolism provide another pathway to expanded consciousness. These patterns, found in both nature and spiritual traditions, resonate with universal truths and archetypal energies. Contemplating a mandala, studying the

Fibonacci sequence, or meditating on the Flower of Life can evoke a sense of unity and harmony, expanding our perception of the cosmos and our place within it.

States of expanded consciousness are also deeply linked to the heart. While the mind seeks logic and analysis, the heart perceives truth through connection and intuition. Practices such as heart-focused meditation or gratitude journaling enhance this connection, creating a sense of openness and compassion that elevates our consciousness.

Service to others is a powerful way to expand consciousness. Acts of kindness, generosity, and empathy dissolve the barriers of the ego, fostering a sense of unity with humanity. Through service, we shift our focus from individual needs to collective well-being, aligning with the interconnected nature of existence and experiencing the joy of contributing to something greater than ourselves.

Challenges and adversity often serve as catalysts for expanding consciousness. Moments of loss, hardship, or uncertainty force us to reevaluate our beliefs, habits, and perspectives. These experiences, while difficult, often lead to profound growth and transformation, revealing the strength and wisdom that lie within.

Creativity and self-expression are integral to the process of expanding consciousness. Artistic pursuits such as painting, music, or writing allow us to channel the energy of the universe, accessing inspiration that transcends the rational mind. These acts of creation connect us to the flow of life, reminding us of the infinite potential within and around us.

The expansion of consciousness also involves integrating the shadow—the parts of ourselves that we suppress or deny. By bringing these aspects into the light with compassion and understanding, we dissolve inner barriers and access deeper layers of awareness. Shadow work, therapy, or journaling can facilitate this process, turning challenges into opportunities for growth.

Communities and collective efforts amplify the expansion of consciousness. Group meditations, spiritual retreats, or global movements for peace and sustainability align individuals with shared intentions, creating powerful fields of energy that elevate collective awareness. These experiences remind us of the profound impact of unity and collaboration.

The expansion of consciousness is not limited to individuals; it is a global phenomenon. Humanity is collectively evolving, as seen in the growing interest in mindfulness, sustainability, and spiritual exploration. This collective awakening reflects a shift toward greater empathy, interconnectedness, and alignment with universal truths.

Stories of expanded consciousness illustrate its transformative power. An individual struggling with a sense of purposelessness finds meaning through meditation and service. A skeptic experiences a profound connection to the universe during a nature retreat, shifting their worldview. A group of strangers comes together for a shared cause, creating a ripple effect of positive change that impacts their community.

Ultimately, the expansion of consciousness is a return to our true nature. It is a journey of remembering the infinite potential and interconnectedness that have always been within us. This process invites us to live with greater awareness, authenticity, and purpose, embracing the mystery and beauty of existence.

In expanding our consciousness, we transcend the limitations of the ego and align with the boundless flow of the universe. This journey transforms not only our inner world but also the world around us, creating a life that reflects the harmony, love, and wisdom of the infinite. By committing to this process, we become co-creators of a reality that honors the interconnectedness of all things, inspiring growth, healing, and transformation on every level.

Chapter 45
Time and the Present Moment

Time is one of the most mysterious and paradoxical aspects of human experience. It governs the rhythms of our lives, yet its nature is elusive. In holistic living, time is more than a linear sequence of events; it is a dynamic flow that connects past, present, and future. By shifting our relationship with time—particularly through the practice of living in the present moment—we can find greater balance, clarity, and fulfillment.

The present moment is the only point of true power and reality. While the mind often oscillates between memories of the past and worries about the future, the present is where life unfolds. It is in the now that we experience the fullness of existence, make conscious choices, and connect with the deeper truths of being. Yet, living fully in the present requires intention and practice, as the distractions of modern life and the habits of the mind often pull us away.

Mindfulness is the foundation of present-moment awareness. This practice involves bringing our full attention to what is happening here and now, without judgment or distraction. Whether focusing on the breath, savoring a meal, or observing the sensations in the body, mindfulness anchors us in the present, enhancing our awareness and appreciation of life's subtleties.

Breathwork is a powerful tool for cultivating presence. The breath is always in the now, serving as a bridge between the body and mind. Simple practices, such as deep diaphragmatic breathing or observing the natural rhythm of the breath, calm the nervous system and draw attention to the present. Over time, these practices create a sense of inner stillness that extends into daily life.

The concept of "psychological time" offers insight into how we experience the present. Psychological time refers to the mental projections that keep us trapped in regret or anticipation, disconnecting us from the here and now. Recognizing these patterns allows us to gently redirect our focus to the present, where clarity and peace reside.

Living in the present does not mean ignoring the past or the future. Instead, it involves integrating them into a balanced perspective. The past holds lessons and memories that shape who we are, while the future represents potential and possibility. By reflecting on the past with gratitude and approaching the future with intention, we honor their roles without losing sight of the present moment.

Gratitude is a transformative practice for embracing the now. By focusing on what is good and meaningful in the present, we shift our perspective from lack to abundance. Simple acts, like journaling about daily blessings or pausing to appreciate the beauty of nature, cultivate a mindset of gratitude that enhances well-being and presence.

The concept of time expands beyond the individual in holistic living. Natural rhythms—such as the cycles of the moon, the seasons, or the flow of day and night—offer a broader perspective on time. Aligning our lives with these rhythms fosters harmony and connection, reminding us of the greater patterns that shape existence.

Rituals create meaningful anchors in time, connecting us to the present while honoring the flow of life. Morning routines, mindful tea ceremonies, or evening reflections provide structure and intention, transforming ordinary moments into sacred practices. These rituals help us pause, reflect, and fully inhabit the present.

Creativity thrives in the present moment. When we engage in activities like painting, writing, or music, we often enter a flow state—a timeless space where the mind is fully immersed in the act of creation. These moments of flow transcend linear time, connecting us to the infinite and opening pathways for inspiration and self-expression.

Nature teaches us profound lessons about time and presence. A tree does not hurry to grow, and a river flows effortlessly toward its destination. Observing these natural processes reminds us to trust the timing of our own lives and to embrace the journey as much as the destination. Time spent in nature naturally grounds us in the present, offering peace and perspective.

Challenges and adversity often draw us into the present with great intensity. Moments of difficulty force us to focus on what is immediate, sharpening our awareness and resilience. These experiences, though painful, often reveal hidden strengths and truths, reminding us of the power of presence in navigating life's storms.

Technology, while a tool for efficiency, often distorts our relationship with time. Constant notifications and endless digital content can fragment our attention, pulling us away from the present. Mindful technology use—such as setting boundaries, taking screen-free breaks, or curating content—helps reclaim focus and presence in a world of distractions.

Meditation on time itself can deepen our understanding of its nature. Practices like reflecting on the impermanence of life or visualizing the flow of time as a river cultivate an appreciation for the fleeting yet precious nature of each moment. This perspective inspires greater mindfulness and intentionality in how we use our time.

Children are natural teachers of present-moment living. Their curiosity, playfulness, and openness embody the essence of being fully present. Spending time with children, engaging in their activities, or simply observing their way of experiencing life offers valuable lessons in reconnecting with the now.

Cultural traditions around the world offer unique insights into time and presence. Indigenous practices, for example, often emphasize the cyclical nature of time, viewing it as a web of interconnected moments rather than a linear progression. These perspectives invite us to reconsider our relationship with time and embrace its fluidity.

Stories of transformation through present-moment awareness illustrate its profound impact. A person overwhelmed by stress discovers peace through daily mindfulness practice. A parent struggling to balance responsibilities reconnects with their child by embracing simple moments of play. An artist facing creative block finds inspiration by immersing themselves in the flow of the present.

Ultimately, the relationship between time and the present moment is a dance of awareness and intention. By honoring the now, we align with the flow of life, experiencing its richness and depth without the weight of past regrets or future anxieties.

In embracing the present moment, we find not only peace but also clarity and purpose. Time becomes a partner rather than an adversary, guiding us toward a life of mindfulness, connection, and meaning. This practice transforms ordinary moments into extraordinary opportunities to live fully, love deeply, and create intentionally, one breath at a time.

Chapter 46
Holistic Leadership

Holistic leadership is an approach to guiding and inspiring others that emphasizes balance, empathy, and alignment with shared values. Unlike traditional leadership, which often focuses on authority, goals, and results, holistic leadership seeks to nurture the whole individual and create environments that foster collective growth and harmony. It is a transformative model that integrates emotional intelligence, spiritual awareness, and practical wisdom, allowing leaders to uplift not only their teams but also their communities and the world at large.

At the heart of holistic leadership is the principle of interconnectedness. A holistic leader recognizes that every decision, interaction, and intention impacts the broader system. By fostering collaboration and unity, they create spaces where individuals feel valued and empowered to contribute their unique talents to a common purpose. This approach shifts leadership from a hierarchy to a partnership, where everyone's voice matters.

Self-awareness is the foundation of holistic leadership. Leaders who understand their strengths, weaknesses, and motivations can approach challenges with clarity and authenticity. Practices like mindfulness, journaling, and self-reflection help leaders stay grounded and aligned with their values. By cultivating inner balance, holistic leaders model the qualities they wish to inspire in others, creating a ripple effect of positivity and purpose.

Empathy is a cornerstone of holistic leadership. Understanding and valuing the perspectives of others builds trust and deepens relationships. Holistic leaders listen actively, seeking to understand not only what is being said but also the emotions and needs underlying the words. This empathetic approach fosters open communication, reduces conflict, and creates a supportive environment where individuals feel seen and heard.

Holistic leadership also emphasizes emotional intelligence—the ability to recognize, manage, and respond to emotions in oneself and others. Leaders with high emotional intelligence navigate challenges with grace, adapt to changing circumstances, and inspire resilience in their teams. This skill is particularly vital in moments of crisis, where emotional steadiness can guide a group through uncertainty with confidence and compassion.

Vision is a defining trait of holistic leaders. They see beyond immediate goals, focusing on long-term impact and alignment with values. Whether leading a team, an organization, or a movement, holistic leaders articulate a vision that inspires and unites others. This vision often extends beyond individual success, encompassing contributions to the greater good, such as sustainability, equity, or community well-being.

Authenticity is another essential quality of holistic leadership. By being genuine and transparent, leaders create an atmosphere of trust and respect. Authenticity invites others to bring their true selves to the table, fostering creativity and collaboration. Holistic leaders understand that vulnerability is not a weakness but a strength that deepens connections and builds trust.

The balance between action and reflection is a key aspect of holistic leadership. While traditional leadership often emphasizes productivity and results, holistic leaders recognize the importance of pausing to assess, reflect, and recalibrate. Practices like mindful decision-making, team retreats, or regular check-ins create opportunities to align actions with intentions, ensuring that progress remains purposeful and sustainable.

Holistic leadership values diversity and inclusivity. By celebrating different perspectives, backgrounds, and strengths, leaders create environments where everyone feels empowered to contribute. This inclusivity not only fosters innovation but also reflects the interconnected nature of holistic principles, where every part of the whole is essential and valued.

One of the challenges of holistic leadership is navigating the tension between personal and collective goals. Leaders must balance the needs of the individual with the objectives of the group, ensuring that neither is sacrificed at the expense of the other. This balance requires clear communication, mutual respect, and a commitment to finding solutions that honor all parties.

Holistic leaders also embrace the role of mentors and guides. They see their position not as one of control but as an opportunity to support and uplift others. By encouraging growth, offering constructive feedback, and celebrating successes, holistic leaders empower those they lead to reach their full potential. This mentorship extends beyond professional development, encompassing emotional and spiritual growth as well.

Sustainability is a core principle of holistic leadership. Leaders who prioritize sustainable practices ensure that their organizations and communities thrive in the long term without depleting resources or harming the environment. This mindset reflects the interconnectedness of all life, emphasizing the importance of stewardship and responsibility in leadership roles.

Holistic leadership also integrates spiritual awareness. While this does not necessarily mean adhering to a specific religion or practice, it involves recognizing the deeper purpose and meaning in leadership. Holistic leaders view their role as a calling to serve, inspire, and contribute to the greater good. Practices like meditation, prayer, or reflection on purpose deepen this spiritual connection, grounding leaders in their values and intentions.

Technology plays a unique role in modern holistic leadership. While it can enhance connection, efficiency, and communication, it also presents challenges, such as burnout and distraction. Holistic leaders model mindful technology use, setting boundaries and encouraging their teams to prioritize well-being over constant availability. This approach fosters balance in an increasingly connected world.

Conflict is an inevitable part of leadership, but holistic leaders approach it as an opportunity for growth and learning. By addressing disagreements with empathy, active listening, and a focus on resolution, they transform conflict into a catalyst for deeper understanding and collaboration. This approach ensures that challenges strengthen rather than divide teams.

Stories of holistic leadership illustrate its transformative power. A leader who prioritizes mental health initiatives creates a workplace culture of resilience and support. A community organizer fosters inclusivity by bringing diverse voices together to address shared challenges. A CEO implements sustainable practices that benefit the environment while inspiring employees to align with values of responsibility and care.

The ripple effect of holistic leadership extends far beyond the immediate group or organization. By fostering balance, empathy, and alignment, holistic leaders contribute to the well-being of communities and even global movements. Their actions inspire others to lead with integrity and purpose, creating a collective shift toward greater harmony and connection.

Ultimately, holistic leadership is about serving as a catalyst for positive change. It is a model that transcends traditional metrics of success, focusing instead on the well-being of individuals, communities, and the planet. By leading with empathy, authenticity, and vision, holistic leaders create environments where growth and harmony flourish.

In embracing holistic leadership, we step into a role of profound responsibility and potential. We become not only guides but also co-creators of a world that reflects the principles of interconnectedness, balance, and shared purpose. This journey of leadership invites us to lead with the heart, inspire with the soul, and act with integrity, transforming both ourselves and the world around us.

Chapter 47
Personal Alchemy

Personal alchemy is the transformative process of turning life's challenges and limitations into opportunities for growth, empowerment, and self-realization. Drawing inspiration from the ancient art of alchemy—where base metals were transformed into gold—this journey involves refining the inner self, dissolving egoic patterns, and embracing the pure potential within. It is a holistic practice that integrates emotional healing, spiritual awakening, and conscious action to create profound change.

The foundation of personal alchemy lies in self-awareness. Transformation begins with an honest examination of one's beliefs, emotions, and habits. This process requires courage, as it often involves confronting aspects of the self that have been hidden or denied. By shining light on these shadows, we begin the work of transmuting them into strengths and wisdom.

One of the most powerful tools in personal alchemy is introspection. Practices such as journaling, meditation, or self-inquiry provide a space for exploring the inner landscape. Questions like, "What patterns are holding me back?" or "What am I being called to learn from this experience?" guide the alchemist inward, uncovering the raw materials for transformation.

Emotional alchemy is a key aspect of this process. Emotions such as fear, anger, or sadness often carry valuable lessons and energies that can be transformed when acknowledged and processed. Techniques like breathwork, emotional release practices, or energy healing allow individuals to move through and release these emotions, uncovering the wisdom and resilience hidden within.

Visualization is another powerful tool for personal alchemy. By imagining oneself as already transformed—stronger, wiser, or more aligned with purpose—we begin to align our thoughts, emotions, and actions with that vision. Visualization acts as a bridge between the current self and the potential self, accelerating the process of transformation.

The stages of personal alchemy often mirror the ancient alchemical process. The first stage, **calcination**, involves breaking down the ego and identifying what no longer serves. This might manifest as the collapse of old beliefs or a life challenge that forces introspection. While this stage can be difficult, it is also the most vital, as it sets the foundation for growth.

The second stage, **dissolution**, is a time of surrender. Here, the alchemist releases attachments and expectations, trusting the process of transformation. In holistic terms, this might involve letting go of a career, relationship, or identity that no longer aligns with one's truth. This phase invites humility and openness, creating space for new possibilities to emerge.

The third stage, **separation**, involves sorting through the elements of the self to identify what is essential. This process requires discernment—deciding which beliefs, habits, or values are worth keeping and which must be discarded. In this stage, the alchemist begins to see their inner gold, the aspects of self that are authentic and aligned with purpose.

The fourth stage, **conjunction**, is the integration of these elements into a cohesive whole. It is a time of alignment, where the alchemist unites the physical, emotional, and spiritual aspects of the self. Practices like mindfulness, yoga, or creative expression help weave these threads together, creating a sense of harmony and balance.

The final stages, **fermentation** and **coagulation**, represent rebirth and embodiment. The alchemist emerges transformed, with a renewed sense of purpose and clarity. This stage is not the end but the beginning of living in alignment with one's highest potential. The lessons and strengths gained through the process become tools for navigating future challenges and inspiring others.

Spirituality often plays a central role in personal alchemy. Connecting with a higher power, whether through prayer, meditation, or nature, provides guidance and support throughout the transformative process. This connection reminds the alchemist that they are not alone, offering a sense of trust in the unfolding journey.

Creativity is another avenue for transformation. Art, music, writing, or movement allow the alchemist to express and process emotions, insights, and shifts. These creative acts are both a reflection of the inner transformation and a catalyst for further growth.

Personal alchemy is not about perfection but integration. It recognizes that challenges are not obstacles but opportunities to refine and grow. Each experience, no matter how difficult, contributes to the creation of the inner gold. This perspective shifts the focus from resistance to curiosity, allowing the alchemist to embrace the process with grace.

Community and connection provide essential support during the alchemical journey. Sharing experiences, seeking guidance from mentors, or joining groups with similar values fosters a sense of belonging and encouragement. These connections remind the alchemist that transformation is a shared human experience, one that unites rather than isolates.

Stories of personal alchemy reveal its transformative power. A person who once struggled with self-doubt discovers their confidence through mindfulness and emotional healing. An individual facing a major life transition learns to release fear and embrace new opportunities with trust. A creative soul transforms past pain into art that inspires and uplifts others.

The ripple effect of personal alchemy extends beyond the individual. As we transform ourselves, we influence those around us, inspiring them to embark on their own journeys of growth.

This collective transformation contributes to the elevation of collective energy, creating a world that reflects harmony, resilience, and possibility.

Ultimately, personal alchemy is a journey of self-realization and empowerment. It invites us to embrace life's challenges as opportunities for growth, to uncover the gold within, and to live with authenticity and purpose.

In stepping into the role of the alchemist, we honor the infinite potential within us. We learn to navigate life's cycles with wisdom and grace, transforming what was once limiting into a source of strength and inspiration. Through personal alchemy, we become not only the creators of our own lives but also contributors to a greater whole, shaping a world of balance, beauty, and possibility.

Chapter 48
Union and Integration

Union and integration are the culmination of holistic living, where the lessons, practices, and transformations experienced throughout the journey come together to create harmony within the self and with the world. This chapter represents the synthesis of all aspects of being—physical, emotional, mental, and spiritual—into a unified and balanced whole. It is a process of bringing together what once seemed fragmented, creating a life that reflects authenticity, purpose, and alignment.

Integration begins with recognizing the interconnectedness of all aspects of our lives. Just as the body, mind, and spirit influence one another, so too do our relationships, environment, and actions contribute to our overall well-being. Union is about honoring these connections, seeing how each element fits into the greater tapestry of our existence, and aligning them with our highest values and intentions.

One of the first steps in integration is reflection. Looking back on the journey—whether through journaling, meditation, or quiet contemplation—reveals the threads that have woven together our experiences. What lessons have emerged? What patterns have been transformed? What truths have been uncovered? Reflection deepens awareness, helping us see the wholeness that has always been present beneath the surface.

Balance is a central theme in integration. It involves finding equilibrium between opposites—activity and rest, effort and surrender, individuality and connection. This balance is not static but dynamic, requiring ongoing awareness and adjustment.

Practices like yoga, Tai Chi, or mindful movement embody this principle, teaching us to flow with the natural rhythms of life.

Union also involves embracing all parts of the self. The holistic journey often brings us face-to-face with the shadow—those aspects of ourselves that we may have denied or judged. Integration requires us to acknowledge these parts with compassion, understanding that they hold valuable lessons and energy. By accepting the entirety of who we are, we create inner harmony and access our full potential.

Spiritual practices play a vital role in fostering union. Meditation, prayer, or rituals that connect us to the divine remind us of our place within the greater whole. These practices align the personal with the universal, deepening our sense of connection to something larger than ourselves. This sense of unity transcends the individual, fostering a profound awareness of interconnectedness with all life.

Integration also extends to relationships. As we cultivate harmony within, we bring that balance into our interactions with others. Practices like active listening, empathetic communication, and setting healthy boundaries create deeper and more authentic connections. Union in relationships involves honoring the uniqueness of each individual while celebrating the shared bond that unites us.

Creativity is another avenue for integration. Artistic expression allows us to process and synthesize our experiences, turning them into something meaningful and beautiful. Whether through painting, writing, music, or dance, creativity bridges the inner and outer worlds, transforming insights into tangible forms that inspire and connect.

Union and integration often involve simplifying life. In a world that values busyness and accumulation, returning to what is essential creates space for clarity and peace. Minimalism, mindful consumption, and intentional living are practical ways to align our outer lives with our inner truths, ensuring that our actions reflect our values.

Nature provides a powerful metaphor for integration. The cycles of growth, decay, and renewal remind us that life is a continuous process of transformation and union. Spending time in nature, observing its harmony and balance, reinforces our connection to the greater whole. Practices like gardening, forest bathing, or simply watching a sunset ground us in this universal truth.

The process of integration is not about perfection but wholeness. It acknowledges that life will always have challenges, changes, and uncertainties. Integration equips us with the tools to navigate these moments with grace and resilience, trusting in our ability to find balance and alignment amidst the flux.

Community and collective connection are integral to union. As individuals integrate their own experiences, they contribute to the harmony of the groups and communities they belong to. Shared practices, rituals, or celebrations strengthen these bonds, creating a sense of belonging and mutual support. Union within the self ripples outward, fostering unity on a larger scale.

Stories of union and integration illustrate their transformative power. A person who once felt fragmented by competing demands finds peace by aligning their actions with their values. A community divided by differences comes together through shared rituals and collective intention. An artist who struggled with self-doubt channels their experiences into a work that inspires others. These stories show how integration creates both personal and collective harmony.

Union also involves aligning with purpose. As we integrate the lessons and transformations of the journey, we gain clarity about what truly matters and how we wish to contribute to the world. This alignment creates a sense of fulfillment and direction, guiding us to live authentically and meaningfully.

The journey of integration is ongoing. Just as the cycles of nature continue endlessly, so too does the process of bringing together new experiences, insights, and challenges. Each stage of life offers opportunities for deeper union, reminding us that growth and harmony are lifelong pursuits.

Ultimately, union and integration reflect the essence of holistic living—a life that honors the interconnectedness of all things and seeks balance, authenticity, and connection. It is a process of coming home to ourselves and to the world, creating a sense of wholeness that radiates outward.

In embracing union, we step into the fullness of who we are. We live with greater presence, compassion, and purpose, knowing that each moment is an opportunity to align with the infinite harmony of existence. Through integration, we create a life that reflects the beauty and unity of the whole, inspiring others to do the same.

Chapter 49
The Holistic Future

The holistic future envisions a world where interconnectedness, balance, and mindfulness are not just ideals but guiding principles for individuals, communities, and global systems. It represents a collective awakening to the importance of harmony—within ourselves, with one another, and with the planet. As humanity evolves, this future invites us to embrace holistic values as the foundation for sustainable growth, innovation, and well-being.

The seeds of the holistic future are already visible in the increasing awareness of practices that prioritize well-being and interconnectedness. Mindfulness, sustainability, and integrative health have moved from the fringes to the mainstream, signaling a shift in collective consciousness. This shift is not merely a trend but a profound realignment with the rhythms of nature and the innate wisdom of humanity.

In this future, health is understood as a dynamic balance of body, mind, and spirit. Holistic health systems integrate ancient practices like acupuncture, Ayurveda, and energy healing with modern medicine, creating a comprehensive approach to well-being. Preventative care becomes a priority, with education and resources empowering individuals to take charge of their health. The focus shifts from treating illness to nurturing vitality and resilience.

Education in the holistic future fosters the development of the whole person. Beyond academic achievement, schools prioritize emotional intelligence, creativity, and spiritual growth. Students are taught to understand their connection to the world and to approach challenges with empathy and innovation. Experiential learning, nature-based education, and mindfulness practices are woven into curricula, creating a generation of leaders who embody holistic principles.

Technology, a defining feature of the modern era, becomes a tool for holistic growth rather than a source of distraction or division. Innovations in artificial intelligence, virtual reality, and renewable energy are designed with mindfulness and sustainability at their core. Technology bridges gaps, enhances well-being, and fosters global collaboration while respecting the balance between digital and natural worlds.

The holistic future also reimagines economics and business. Organizations prioritize purpose over profit, adopting models that value people, planet, and prosperity equally. Conscious capitalism, circular economies, and regenerative practices become the norm. Employees are supported through wellness programs, flexible work environments, and opportunities for personal growth, fostering a culture of balance and fulfillment.

Sustainability is a cornerstone of the holistic future. Humanity recognizes its role as a steward of the planet, embracing practices that restore ecosystems and honor natural resources. Renewable energy, organic farming, and zero-waste initiatives are no longer exceptional but standard. Communities thrive through localized, eco-conscious practices, demonstrating that sustainability and prosperity can coexist.

Spirituality in the holistic future is inclusive and expansive. It transcends dogma, encouraging individuals to explore their connection to the divine in ways that resonate personally. Practices like meditation, breathwork, and ritual are embraced universally, fostering inner peace and collective harmony. This spiritual awakening deepens humanity's sense of purpose and unity, reminding us of our shared journey.

Art and culture flourish in the holistic future, serving as expressions of the interconnectedness and creativity that define this era. Music, visual arts, and storytelling bridge divides, inspiring empathy and understanding across cultures. Festivals and gatherings celebrate diversity while honoring the shared values of community and connection.

Communities in the holistic future are built on collaboration and mutual support. Urban areas are redesigned with green spaces, shared resources, and sustainable infrastructure. Rural areas thrive through initiatives that value biodiversity and local traditions. Technology connects these communities without diminishing the importance of face-to-face relationships, creating a global network of support and innovation.

Global challenges—climate change, inequality, and political unrest—are addressed through collective action rooted in holistic principles. Governments and organizations prioritize long-term solutions over short-term gains, guided by values of equity, sustainability, and peace. Collaboration replaces competition, fostering a world where humanity works together for the greater good.

The holistic future also honors the wisdom of indigenous cultures and ancient traditions. Practices that have sustained communities for centuries—such as rituals, storytelling, and deep connection to the land—are integrated into modern systems, providing a balance of innovation and tradition. This respect for ancestral knowledge enriches the holistic vision, reminding humanity of its roots.

Individual transformation is at the heart of the holistic future. As more people embrace mindfulness, self-awareness, and healing, they contribute to the collective energy of growth and harmony. This ripple effect creates a feedback loop, where personal and collective evolution reinforce one another. Every act of kindness, every moment of presence, becomes a building block for a more compassionate world.

The holistic future is not without challenges. Resistance to change, fear of the unknown, and deeply ingrained systems can slow progress. However, these challenges are met with resilience, creativity, and collaboration. Humanity learns to see obstacles as opportunities for growth, transforming adversity into wisdom and strength.

Stories of transformation illuminate the path to the holistic future. Communities devastated by environmental disasters rebuild using sustainable practices, becoming models of resilience. Leaders once driven by profit discover purpose in serving others, inspiring industries to adopt conscious practices. Individuals who felt disconnected and lost find meaning through holistic healing, contributing their gifts to the world.

The holistic future is not a distant ideal but a choice we make in the present. Every mindful action, every step toward balance and connection, brings this vision closer to reality. By embracing holistic principles today, we lay the foundation for a world where harmony, well-being, and unity are not aspirations but lived experiences.

In this future, humanity thrives not in isolation but in collaboration—with one another, with nature, and with the universe. The journey of transformation becomes a collective endeavor, a shared story of awakening and integration. The holistic future reminds us that we are not separate from the world but an integral part of its unfolding, capable of co-creating a reality that reflects the beauty and interconnectedness of life itself.

In choosing this path, we honor our deepest truths and highest aspirations. The holistic future invites us to live with intention, love with depth, and create with purpose, forging a world that is not only sustainable but also profoundly fulfilling—a future where the harmony of the whole is celebrated, cherished, and continuously renewed.

Epilogue

What is essential is rarely found in the noise of the world but in the spaces of silence and presence. Walking the path of holistic living reveals that balance is not a fixed state but a constant dance between the parts that form the whole. Mind, body, emotions, and the surrounding environment are not separate entities but aspects of a single flow.

The principles shaping this understanding are not new; they transcend time, sustained by traditions and validated by modern experience. The harmony of living begins with small daily choices that honor the interconnectedness of all things. From the simplicity of an intentional breath to the impact of conscious actions on the collective, each gesture carries the seed of transformation.

The core of holism is not perfection but presence. The ability to view life's cycles with acceptance allows for deeper engagement with the present moment. Every challenge becomes an opportunity for learning; every joy, a celebration of the unity underlying diversity.

On the journey to holistic living, self-awareness emerges as an essential tool. Observing thoughts, emotions, and habits without judgment reveals patterns that can be adjusted to align intentions and actions. This continuous practice of refinement not only uplifts the individual but also enriches the collective fabric of life.

Reconnecting with nature is one of the pillars of this path. Whether in the vastness of a forest or the simple act of touching the soil, nature reminds us of the innate connection between humanity and the planet. In this reconnection, it becomes clear that personal well-being is intrinsically linked to the Earth's balance.

From this perspective, living holistically is not a distant goal but a daily commitment. Each moment offers an opportunity to act with intention, cultivate harmony, and honor the web of interdependencies that sustains existence. The path is ongoing, and every step is an act of conscious creation.

The legacy of this vision does not lie in grand changes but in the constancy of small actions. True transformation happens when the ordinary is lived with extraordinary awareness, when life ceases to be divided into fragments and becomes an integrated whole.

May the understanding of the deep connections between all things continue to guide every choice. May the journey never cease to surprise. And may balance, even in its fluidity, always remain a living possibility.

www.ingramcontent.com/pod-product-compliance
Lightning Source LLC
LaVergne TN
LVHW040052080526
838202LV00045B/3591